Praise for the Authors

'Having witnessed Yasmin's growth and commitment to health as a way of life for the past twenty years, I know that her book will help many more bodies believe that that's the best place for a soul to live.'

Salman Khan, actor

'I realized after reading the script of *Cocktail* that it would be a unique film in my career. I remember telling myself that it was a very special role and I had to make it exceptional. The character needed me to work on my physical self. When I spoke to people, they said, "But why do you need to work out? You're already so fit and athletic!" But I looked at myself in the mirror and knew I could do something different. That difference was Yasmin Karachiwala.

'Yasmin introduced me to Pilates. Within a couple of sessions I was addicted! I could actually see my body transform. Pilates has made me realize how we neglect our core and also how important breathing correctly is. It helps me focus! It helps me on a stressful day!

'Being an athlete has taught me that it's not the number of hours you spend in the gym, but the quality of workout time that you put in. Even just a 20–30-minute session with the right focus and dedication can make a difference. Fitness has to become a part of one's lifestyle.

'I believe that physical fitness is a combination of the mind and the body. Working on your mind is as important as working on your body. And with Yasmin, it's always the perfect combination of both.

'Yasmin is not just my trainer. She is my friend first . . . my confidante. She makes you believe that you are capable of achieving the impossible. She has a constant desire to keep improving her craft and her techniques. She has an endless desire to learn, to grow and be the best! For me, she is already the best.'

Deepika Padukone, actor

'I first met Yasmin Karachiwala at a party. I had gained quite a bit of weight and she told me she could help me lose it. At first, we started with functional training as she was still setting up her Pilates studio; as soon as it was ready, we moved on to Pilates.

'The best thing about Pilates is that it is a healthy, gentle and sustainable approach to fitness, based on strengthening and stretching your muscles. Your body feels wonderfully realigned and refreshed. Often, high-intensity CrossFit or functional training (which is very good when you have a specific or quick target to achieve) can be very strenuous on the body. This is especially true if you have any joint or back issues. Pilates is a very gentle way of training your muscles without further injury to yourself.

'Pilates also helps improve your posture. Today, it continues to be embraced by professional dancers. This assures you of the effectiveness of Pilates, as dancers put their bodies through a lot of strain. Pilates can realign any misbalances that occur. During intense physical preparation for films like *Dhoom 3*, and songs such as 'Sheila ki Jawaani', Pilates has always been an integral part of my training.

'Yasmin has a wonderfully positive attitude at all times and she makes training fun. She'll often adapt or change our training sessions according to my mood or energy level. Often, when I have intense periods of training, like before *Dhoom 3*, she will train with me, as in, do each exercise along with me because I don't like doing it on my own. She's very passionate about her clients achieving their results.

'I always feel better when I'm healthy and fit! I believe that there are no shortcuts to becoming fit. If you want to be fit and healthy or if you want to correct an injury, you have to put in the time. It is important to be regular and incorporate Pilates as part of your lifestyle.'

Katrina Kaif, actor

'My first squat, my first lunge and my first bicep curl—that's where my journey with Yasmin began. From teaching walking-lunges in her living room—her gym about fifteen-odd years ago—to becoming a woman who is a superstar herself and the reason why all of us are looking our best, Yasmin is the soundest mind on fitness. She is someone I admire for her time management—for giving equal importance to all the lovely superstars by giving each one their required time as per their body type. That's her finest professional quality. To me, she will always be a friend first and then a fitness guide. Our journey is forever and with Pilates, our new friend, it has just begun. Here's to you, Yasmin—to the most well-deserved success story, and to many more amazing and insightful books to come.'

Kareena Kapoor, actor

'Once upon a time, about one year ago, I was having an anxiety attack. I had one month to look sexy in a bikini. I had lost a whopping amount of weight and was beginning to look like a boy! Which, for obvious reasons, is not sexy at all!

'Then, my very efficient manager hooked me up with another very efficient human being. Enter Yasmin Karachiwala. I think it's safe to say the first time I met Yas, I was a bit scared (you would be too if you had been there). Fluorescent clothes, sprinting away on the cross trainer wearing the ATS (Altitude Training Systems) machine, which kind of makes you look like a monster or robot (which, by the way, is now my favourite machine—great for burning fat). However, within a month of training with Yas, or even less actually, it's safe to say I was in love. From not being able to stand straight with my two feet on the ground, she now has me doing squats on the flat side of the BOSU ball. Okay, that still sounds complicated. Even though I had been working out before I met her, the gym was always a burden for me. A place I had to push myself to go to. But here, it's the other way around. I have to push myself to *not* go to the gym sometimes.

'Apart from Yasmin, there was something else that I fell in love with—Pilates. At first, I was confused! I had done a couple of sessions before, but that was ages ago, and I was probably sleeping through the class. But this time, Pilates seemed very exotic. A special room at Yasmin's studio, Body Image, is dedicated only to Pilates, and contains all the necessary and extremely fascinating Pilates equipment. We have the Reformer, which is multifaceted—you can use it for three different types of workouts. Then there's the

Wunda Chair, which is as fun as the name suggests, and then comes my favourite, which is CoreAlign—again, as the name suggests, the best thing for your core (also known as the stomach, which you will want to show off in a bikini or a lehenga!).

'I have only been doing it for eight months and I've seen a massive change in my core strength, so imagine what I'll feel like when I do it for longer! Pilates is all about hand-eye coordination and focus. You have to mentally be very present to do it right. There is not a single point where your core is at ease; you have to keep it activated at all times, but that comes with lots of practice. I am an impatient person but with Yas, I've learnt how to be patient and strengthen my body for the long run rather than lose five kilos in a month, which will eventually come back after one holiday. She doesn't help you just lose your weight; she helps you develop and maintain a healthy and fit lifestyle; so in the long run, when you do lose the weight, it stays that way.

'What I love the most is that I enjoy my workouts at Body Image. It's not just the same thing over and over again. It's almost like a school, where you move from workout to workout and graduate to different levels, and with this, your strength, and obviously your body, are changing and improving. With Pilates, all the workouts and exercises have these interesting, quirky names. And as Yasmin once told me, Pilates is all about the imagination as well. "Imagine there's a bowl of water on your stomach"; "Roll the marble"; "Shine your chest" and my favourite, "Look at the horizon", which basically means, "Alia, stop looking at yourself in the mirror."

'The kind of erratic lifestyle that I lead, it gets hard to stick to just one timing sometimes. But with her complete focus and dedication, she will come any time—be it 6 a.m. or 10 p.m. But I must mention, I get a firing every time I'm late! In short, if you haven't already understood the pros and pros of Body Image, you must be really slow. Put on your gym clothes and shoes (make sure you match and colour-coordinate them—another thing I've learnt from Yas) and go to Yasmin's Body Image now, now, now!'

Alia Bhatt, actor

'Whatever I say about Yasmin will never be enough. She is one of the most dedicated, sincere, hard-working and affable people I know. Her knowledge about training, workouts, nutrition, etc. is so vast and precise. She makes going to the gym so much fun. She has truly changed the game. Thank you so much for introducing Pilates to me. It has changed my body and, more importantly, my life. You truly are an inspiration and we love you.'

Malaika Arora Khan, actor

'I heard much talk of Pilates in various social conversations, but I stayed away . . . till I met the relentless, persistent, but immensely affable, Yasmin. This may sound wrong, but she made me feel parts of my body that I didn't know existed. This will sound even more wrong but she made me stretch in directions I never had before. Along with Pilates, she introduced me to ATS, which makes you feel like you've come from a good run in Ladakh without actually having been there. Her constant follow-ups make me feel like I now have two mothers in the world . . . While that thought can be annoying at times, it's tremendously comforting as well. So, has Yasmin been responsible for making me love my enemy? Not entirely . . . but because of her, I am civil with it today.'

Karan Johar, film-maker

'I was diagnosed with a bulging disc. It was a very confusing time for me—"Wear a brace", "Don't wear a brace", "Your muscles should work", "Sit upright", "Don't sit for too long", "Stretch your back", "Rest your back", "Physio helps", "Yoga heals" . . . blah blah blah blah. I was prepping for my film and was slated to travel for one month looking for locations. I was in pain and often wondering when my L4-L5 was planning to pop out and pay me a visit. I spoke to Yasmin, who introduced me to Pilates. Slowly, I became strong and my core grew stronger. Pilates is a part of my life now and I can't do without it. My back is in great shape and the rest of me seems to be catching up too.'

Zoya Akhtar, director

'There are days when my body just feels sore and tired, and doing a session of Pilates just stretches it out and makes me feel great and rejuvenated. I look forward to my sessions with Yasmin. She pushes me to do better every day and the results are clearly visible. Plus, it really is motivating when you have a trainer as fit and gorgeous as Yasmin—it just makes you want to work that much harder to get a body that you will love in the years to come.'

Ileana D'Cruz, actor

'Pilates gives you so much body awareness, it really helps you to connect your body, mind and soul. It gives you tremendous core strength and flexibility, and it's extremely challenging! I'm actually miserable if I am unable to work out! I feel fitter, happier and stronger whenever I practise Pilates and it is a form of exercise I recommend to everyone, especially anyone with injuries! Thank you, Yasmin, for making me feel and look so fit and fabulous.'

Sophie Choudry, actor–singer

'Yasmin is the kind of trainer whom you love and dread at the same time. You love her for how you look once she is done with you, and you dread her when she is training with you as she pushes you to your limit. I love her attitude at work and her attention to detail. She is undoubtedly the best in the business and takes extra care if you have an injury. She has a vast amount of knowledge and experience and has been in the fitness business for as long as I can remember. Don't get deceived by her pretty face, as underneath, she is tough as nails. Go to her if you are willing to work hard and love your body. You will never be disappointed.'

Preity Zinta, actor

'Working with Yasmin really helped me fix a lot of issues with my posture, flexibility and balance. Core strength and stability are vital for action sequences and dancing, and that's where I really saw a difference in my capabilities.'

Imran Khan, actor

'I went to Yasmin with a couple of injuries, and she made them worse and then refused to refund my money. Haha! On a serious note—Yasmin is one of the most incredible trainers. Her approach to fitness is unique and holistic. Working with her helped me take my fitness to a new level and look at training in a whole new light.'

Kunal Kapoor, actor

'Adding the Pilates workout to my routine of strength and conditioning, along with training on the field for cricket, has benefited me. Thank you, Yasmin, for making the Pilates workouts fun by adding variety.'

Zaheer Khan, cricketer

'I've never known anyone who is as passionate as Yasmin when it comes to fitness. She's always travelling to push herself and learn newer techniques, which all her clients are excited to learn when she returns. There's never a dull moment at Body Image. It's the thing I look forward to every morning and the sense of achievement you get after that workout, motivates you to conquer the rest of your day.'

Kiara Advani, actor

'Pilates is my Monday, Wednesday and Friday must! It involves strengthening, firming, lengthening and healing one's body to its best shape. Five years ago, my knees refused to work and cardio was ruled out. I was looking for the perfect complement to yoga, which I've done most of my life, and Yasmin, my little body goddess, introduced me to this perfect art called Pilates. I cannot thank her enough! Body Image, for me, is just the best.'

Rhea Pillai, former model

'Pilates is the best and definitely the most fun type of workout for me. In only five sessions, I can feel a definite change in my body! I have tried many workouts in the course of my career, but I have never seen such quick results as when training with Yasmin. My arms and legs are super toned and my core muscles have become really strong. I feel fit, beautiful and ready to shoot! Yasmin is like a genie doing wonders.'

Evelyn Sharma, actor

'For me, Pilates means Yasmin Karachiwala. She introduced me to Pilates when I had no idea what it was. I'm thankful to her for doing so because it really did wonders for me. It not only helped me sculpt my body but also taught me the importance of having a strong core and a well-aligned body. I wish her all the very best for the book and I'm happy that it will help a lot of people understand and enjoy the benefits of Pilates.'

Zareen Khan, actor

'As an actor, I've always been very particular about keeping myself in shape. I've turned to Zeena Dhalla over the years as someone who can teach me about my core, and how to keep the correct muscles in shape to stay injury-free. Zeena brings to the world of Pilates her attention to detail, a clear passion for success and a commitment to excellence. I've known Zeena for over twenty years, and I have been consistently impressed with her ability to help her clients achieve their goals, in a gentle, but tough-love way. I'm thrilled that the world will get to read the myriad of her teachings through the book *Sculpt and Shape: The Pilates Way*. This book will not only help the reader become more aware of his or her body, it will offer invaluable education on the proper exercises to look and feel better from the inside out.'

Kristofer McNeeley,
actor, Hollywood executive

'When I think Pilates, I think of Yasmin Karachiwala. She brings a new dimension to Pilates, making it fun and enjoyable whilst at the same time ensuring one achieves one's ultimate health goals. It's no wonder that the Bollywood and sporting elite are seen flocking to her. Here's wishing you all the best for the book *Sculpt and Shape*. I'm sure the readers will get a glimpse of the magic you make during your classes.'

Kinita Kadakia Patel,
sports nutrition consultant

'Pilates—a sports physiotherapist's best friend. Thank you, Yasmin, for embracing the concept, perfecting the techniques and delivering such an important component of everyday life to so many. A must for every sportsperson, gym junkie, couch potato and desk-bound individual to get the best out of their professional and social lives. A fitness regime beyond all others.'

John Gloster, sports physiotherapist

'This book talks about crucial things like how to stand, walk and breathe, and before you say, "Oh! I know that", stop and read the book, and you will be surprised how little you actually know. Reading the book is only half the job. After finishing the book, begin the practice of Pilates. This book is to inspire you to practise. In fact, as I have told Yasmin, the book should have been titled *Zen and the Art of Pilates* because Yasmin is like a Zen master when she is practising Pilates. And just as Zen is best learnt from a Zen master, Pilates is best learnt from arguably India's best, Yasmin Karachiwala. And after you learn from the book, pray you get lucky like me, and she trains you one day.'

Ridham Desai,
managing director, Morgan Stanley, India

'I have had the privilege of knowing Zeena for thirteen years. Throughout that time, Zeena has continually found ways to educate and expose people to a healthy and balanced lifestyle. *Sculpt and Shape* is more than an exercise and diet book. It is a way of living, a way of thinking and a way of moving. When reading, I found myself being immediately mindful of my posture, sitting or standing. The Pilates programmes are so straightforward and understandable. I am so proud of my friend Zeena for creating this simple yet profound book of posture and well-being. May this book inspire us all to live our best life.'

Jennifer Pearlstein,
Body Arts and Science International, Pilates senior faculty

'Being a golf professional, I have worked with various fitness coaches. Zeena is among the best! She is a great communicator, she is knowledgeable and she pays great attention to detail; if I perform any exercise incorrectly, she corrects my form and I repeat the exercise, recruiting the correct muscles. Pilates is a powerful exercise regimen, and I hope her book will inspire others to integrate precise, posture-focused workouts into their routines.'

Michelle Dúbe,
Ladies Professional Golf Association,
master golf professional

SCULPT
AND SHAPE

SCULPT AND SHAPE

THE PILATES WAY

YASMIN KARACHIWALA | ZEENA DHALLA

Maulie –
Enjoy getting
aligned!

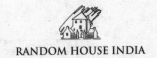

RANDOM HOUSE INDIA

Published by Random House India in 2015

Second impression in 2015

Random House Publishers India Pvt. Ltd
7th Floor, Infinity Tower C, DLF Cyber City
Gurgaon – 122002
Haryana

Random House Group Limited
20 Vauxhall Bridge Road
London SW1V 2SA
United Kingdom

978 81 8400 597 4

The views and opinions expressed in this book are the authors'
own and the facts are as reported by them which have been
verified to the extent possible, and the publishers are not in
any way liable for the same.

Please consult a physician before beginning
any exercise regimen.

Typeset in Sabon by Manipal Digital Systems, Manipal

Printed at Replika Press Pvt. Ltd, India

A PENGUIN RANDOM HOUSE COMPANY

*To our fathers for encouraging us to be strong,
independent women.
To our mothers for showing us how.*

CONTENTS

FOREWORD

Both the authors are true professionals and masters of the art and science of fitness in general, and Pilates in particular. Read this book and you will understand why. They have covered all the essentials of living a fit life—from posture to the exercises, and everything in between.

This unique concept was brought to the world by its founder Joseph Pilates and developed in the early 1900s. It is practised widely in the USA and Europe. It was Yasmin (the pioneer of Pilates), the only BASI-certified trainer in our country, who had the foresight to bring it to our subcontinent.

On reading this book, I am quite amazed at the many similarities between Pilates and martial arts. They include postural control, muscular endurance, strength and flexibility with a very strong core. The authors have also given an entire chapter to breathing, and rightly so. Breathing correctly is the essence of life and more so in performing any type of physical activity.

Their chapter on nutrition is well postulated and gives a whole new meaning to what, when and even how to eat. It makes for easy understanding and easier implementation, with small but essential changes in nutrition.

Being fit enables you to do all that you want to—climb a mountain, take part in a marathon or go skydiving. It also enhances your self-esteem and confidence, and is proven to give you a long and healthy life. All this is possible if you follow the advice of Joseph Pilates, through his ardent advocates, Yasmin and Zeena.

I am positive that it will help all those who follow this fitness road to meet life's maladies and stress far better than ever before.

Sensei B. Mistry
Chief Instructor, IOGKF India
Post-Exercise Rehabilitative Specialist, AFPA

INTRODUCTION

How did I, an Indian girl born and raised in the good old United States of America, manage to write a book with Yasmin Karachiwala, the top fitness instructor in Mumbai? It all started with one simple phone call in the year 2006. Yasmin had travelled all the way from India to Orange County, California, to learn about a new fitness regimen called Pilates. For her certification programme, she was referred to the women's gym, which I owned at the time, to take some Pilates mat classes. Upon meeting, we hit it off right away, and a true friendship developed.

After a few weeks of interaction in California, we discovered that there couldn't be two more similar women who were raised on opposite ends of the globe. My family was of Indian descent but immigrated to the US before I was born. I am as American as it gets. Yasmin is a true-blood Indian, but often travels to the US to take advantage of the educational opportunities in the fitness industry. What is common between us is that we both share an extreme passion for helping change lives.

For both of us, being fit isn't just about a flat stomach or slimmer thighs—athough that's a wonderful by-product of getting fit. Being fit also means being mentally strong, feeling more confident and achieving every goal in life that we set forth to achieve. Being a fitness trainer means inspiring people, educating clients and being examples of the change that we want to see in them.

My Fitness Story

I entered the fitness industry in my late twenties, after a few years in an unsatisfactory career—I had been a producer in Hollywood. I was out of shape and unhappy, overweight and sloppy. One day, while driving to the job that made me rather miserable, I heard an advertisement for a marathon-training programme. I thought, 'Wow! I wonder if I could ever run a marathon!' I joined the training programme. Every week, we added more miles to our run, and every week, I ran farther and longer than I could have ever imagined.

I felt powerful, I lost weight, I felt confident and I accomplished things in my personal and professional life that I didn't expect. The experience of training for this marathon changed my body, but more importantly, it changed my life. Every week, I accomplished a new goal, running farther than I ever had before. By the end of the experience, I decided that fitness needed to be my new career. I earned my first certification to be a personal trainer at the National Academy of Sports Medicine (NASM), and eventually decided to own my own women's gym, the Athletic Club for Women. It was in this business that I discovered my passion for Pilates, and completed the Body Arts and Sciences International (BASI) Pilates certification course in 2004. At the time, Pilates had only begun to grow popular in the US, and our studio was the first in the area to introduce the concept of Pilates equipment classes for small groups.

In 2007, I decided to sell my women's gym to become an adoptive mom. I travelled to India for the first time ever, to pick up my daughter from an orphanage in Kolkata. Yasmin was there for me along the way, introducing me to my Indian heritage and becoming an auntie to my new daughter. After a few years of stay-at-home motherhood, I opened a new studio, Vertical Pilates (the first vertical-only Pilates studio in the US) in 2012. It had always been a dream of mine to bring more postural alignment and awareness to the art of Pilates, and my studio in California reflects this dream. I have been lucky to develop a strong reputation in my area, having written for and contributed to numerous local websites, magazines and TV shows.

My Life Story

I grew up as an only child with loving parents who put an emphasis on faith and education. The best thing about my parents was that despite their wish for me to be a lawyer, they allowed me to choose the career I wanted. When, at the age of twenty-eight, I wanted to drop everything and become a personal trainer, they supported me and encouraged me to become the best personal trainer I could ever be. I have also been blessed to marry the first man I ever dated and loved, my high-school sweetheart Azeem Dhalla—a man who still supports me in whatever endeavour I embark on.

My journey to motherhood was challenging and our decision to travel to India and adopt a child, however scary and courageous, is again a testament to the love and support in my life. It has been the greatest challenge with the biggest reward, and it has completely changed me from the inside out.

I now live my life with more patience, compassion, empathy and gratitude. I genuinely think I could not have written this book had it not been for the patience and perseverance I learnt from being a mother on a difficult journey.

My Inspiration

In my Pilates career, my first instructor, Rael Isocawitz, shaped my perspective and taught me how to never compromise on the movement. My friend Jennifer Pearlstein has always inspired me with her unwavering loyalty, dedication and commitment to our art.

In life, I am inspired by those who overcome adversity with a relentless pursuit of positivity.

Lastly, I am inspired by a world that somehow brought me together with my beautiful daughter. She challenges me to my core, and she inspires me to do better and be better in everything I do.

                                                    Zeena Dhalla

Believe it or not, I got involved in the fitness industry by fluke! I was extremely lazy back in the day and would only exercise when forced to. In school, I'd participate in just a handful of sporting activities like the march-past, javelin and shot-put. When I was eighteen years old, my life changed when my best friend dragged me to a local gym to sign up so that she could get a discount on a two-for-one deal. Reluctantly, I agreed.

During our first session at the gym, I sauntered past the machines and the weights to the aerobics room, thinking to myself, 'How difficult can this be?' I couldn't have been more wrong! I spent that entire class feeling like a klutz, very clumsy in my movements. I made an utter fool of myself that day.

Embarrassed by the way I had performed, I returned to the class day after day to improve my skills. I dislike failing to perform well in the things that I try; I therefore worked very hard to master all the aerobic routines. Gradually, I progressed from the back of the class to the front, and eventually became the best student. One fateful morning, my aerobics instructor called in sick and asked me to substitute for her.

Surprised and thrilled at the opportunity, I agreed, and soon realized that teaching aerobics class was one of the most amazing experiences of my life so far. Encouraged by the instructor, I decided to pursue fitness as a career. I didn't just want to copy Jane Fonda routines and teach classes; I wanted to have knowledge of the correct techniques. Two years later, I went to the United States and earned my certification as a group fitness trainer from the American Council on Exercise (ACE). I started my career as a group step-aerobics instructor and, after a few years, went and earned my certification as a personal trainer. Sometimes, I find it amazing what destiny has in store for you; this was the best career choice for me, since I'm completely passionate about fitness.

In 2006, I felt the need to learn something new, so I searched extensively and finally decided to go to the US and learn how to teach Pilates (BASI certification). I found that it was the answer my clients were looking for to get washboard abs. Of course, I learnt that the benefits go far beyond just having a slim midsection.

My first celebrity client was Kareena Kapoor. This was ten years ago when my studio was inside my home. She heard about me from some friends and wanted to try out a class. As time passed, seeing Kareena achieve her desired results, other celebrities started to trickle into my studio as well. My popularity grew tenfold after I started my Pilates studio, as I found that Pilates fine-tuned the body in the perfect way, and helped celebrities look stunning on screen. More importantly, since their bodies took a beating from dancing and stunt work, Pilates aligned them so that they didn't have any injuries thereafter. My celebrity clients include Deepika Padukone, Katrina Kaif, Kareena Kapoor, Alia Bhatt, Ileana D'Cruz, Sophie Choudry, Malaika Arora Khan, Preity Zinta, Zareen Khan, Shazahn Padamsee and Kiara Advani. I have also trained cricketers like Zaheer Khan and Ajit Agarkar.

My Life Story

I grew up in a nuclear family with my parents and one older brother. Since I had green eyes and looked different from my family, my brother would tease me and say I was adopted. This traumatized me and I would cry for hours. I despised my brother growing up because he always excelled in everything he took on, from schooling to sports. I, however, was too naughty to focus on any one thing.

When I decided to become an instructor and made plans to go to the US to study and train, he pointed out that I would just be wasting my parents' money and my time yet again, and, like everything else in my past, wouldn't complete it. This time his words really hurt me and I was determined to prove him wrong. In my certification programme, I got a rude shock;

I was expecting it to be more practical and less theoretical. The theory was not easy, especially since I didn't come from a science background. But I had a point to prove, so for six months I worked really hard, completed my certification and came home a trained instructor. The person who was made happiest by my achievement was my brother. In that moment, I realized that this was the reason he had constantly taunted me; he wanted me to abandon my laziness and realize my full potential. He knew that negative criticism would make me want to prove him wrong, and in the process, my brother brought out the best in me. My brother has always been, and will always be, my biggest supporter.

Believe it or not, I met my husband by fluke too; an uncle insisted I meet this really nice boy he knew, who he thought would be the perfect match for me. Once again, reluctantly, I agreed to meet this man and it turned out to be the second-best fluke of my life. We took an instant liking to each other on our very first meeting and met every single day after that until we got married in 1993. He is the most impatiently patient man, and has been extremely supportive of my every decision and allowed me to pursue my career. I couldn't have been more blessed and I thank God every day.

My sons are the reason I broke the trend of training people in their houses. When I started personal training they were toddlers, two years apart, and I felt the need to be around them even while I worked. So I started calling clients home and converted one room into a little studio. This way, I could work and be around for the times when my boys were ready to chop each other up. Thanks to them, I made a decision that has led me to where I am today.

Though my sons are not very happy about it now, one of the perks of having me as their mother is that they don't have a choice but to be fit.

My Inspiration

My biggest inspiration is Sensei Pervez Mistry, hailed as the father of karate in India. I first met him in 2004 (I had been an aerobics instructor for three years) when a friend suggested we start weight training. Although I was pretty happy with the way I looked until I met Sensei, he looked at me and commented that though I appeared slim, I had a lot of fat. I was shocked to learn that my fat percentage was pretty high. I trained under Sensei for ten years and from him I learnt the most important rule of fitness: never compromise on form while doing any exercise.

In 2006, when I went to Orange County for my Pilates training, I met another person who inspired me just as much as Sensei. Rael Isacowitz gave me my first introduction to Pilates. Rael reinforced the rule of always working with the right form and taught me that instructing clients to achieve proper alignment can be a true passion.

I am a running enthusiast and have run four half-marathons. My philosophy stems from my passion and enthusiasm for fitness. Enjoyment is key; fitness for me is all about fun. You have to incorporate fitness into your lifestyle. If you don't enjoy it, you will not pursue it as a lifestyle, so you need to find the type of exercise and activities that make you feel good. What works for me may not necessarily work for you.

Yasmin Karachiwala

WHY THIS BOOK?

We've always been astounded by how we think the same, work the same and train the same, despite being across the world from each other. We wanted to do business together, years ago, but the distance (over 12,000 kilometres) was overwhelming. Then the opportunity to write a book came along, and when we were asked to jump at it, we asked, 'How high?'

Writing a book was the next big challenge for both of us. It takes patience, perseverance, focus and commitment. Wait—isn't this also what you need to achieve fitness goals and get into shape? If we can stay committed to our fitness regime, then we can do anything, right? This book is proof of it.

We've overcome over twelve hours of time-zone difference, constant scheduling challenges and spotty Internet calls, and managed to get our words down on paper. We are moms and business owners, and busier than we've ever been, but somehow we've managed to complete a book that we are both extremely proud of.

We took the same Pilates certification course two years apart from one another, and since that experience, we have both gone on to develop new ideas and concepts with regard to what we think is the best of Pilates. We've taken a plethora of certification courses in the Pilates realm and we both now run certification courses ourselves. We build on the framework Pilates has given us to grow our businesses and train our clients the best way we know. Now we want to share this knowledge with you.

This isn't your normal exercise book with pages of pictures you can mimic mindlessly. Our goal is to teach you the science, the reasoning and the methodology of how to perform Pilates properly. We've made some changes to the original Pilates repertoire, and we will educate you on why we made these changes. We will teach you about your own body, your posture, why it's important and how to change it. We spend a lot of time discussing posture, since proper posture is the key to physical longevity and injury prevention. We will also delve into how to eat, sit, stand, walk, sleep, breathe and think.

Yes, we love being bossy; it's what we do for a living. Every day, when we see the changes in our client's lives, we understand that we were meant to do this for a living. Sometimes, we have to pinch ourselves because we can hardly believe we are lucky enough to be living our passion on a daily basis.

If you read every page in this book, and we hope you do, we know that you will become inspired by the Pilates methodology like we have. Much like yoga is a way of life, Pilates is the same. Once you learn how to truly engage your core and work from your centre, there is no going back. Your body will change, your mind will focus and your life will begin to move from your centre. Once the body has engaged in a regular Pilates programme for a few months, the muscles will not forget this, and it will positively impact the way you move for the rest of your life.

We encourage you to read every chapter and try every exercise. Do the postural assessments and practise the breathing. Learn how to do things properly, because with proper movement comes proper results.

India has seen several changes in the fitness industry's trends, but it has yet to fully embrace the world of Pilates. In the United States, Pilates has proven that it has value as a long-term solution to everyday fitness problems. It's now time for India to see and understand that fitness can be fully achieved with the precision, control and concentration that Pilates develops.

HOW TO USE THIS BOOK

We assume your reason for picking up this book is to get stronger, become more flexible or lose some weight. Perhaps your goal is all of the above, and Pilates caught your attention and intrigues you. If so, you've picked up the correct book.

Before you jump to Chapter 8, where we list a majority of the exercises, we highly recommend you read the other chapters, which will prepare you for the workout component of the book.

In Chapter 1, you will learn about Joseph Pilates and how he developed his revolutionary form of exercise. You will learn the difference between mat Pilates and equipment Pilates. You will walk away from this chapter with a solid understanding of the principles of Pilates and how you can integrate them into your Pilates practice. This is extremely important before embarking on your first workout.

Chapter 2 spends a good amount of time helping you understand posture, your muscles and how it all works together. We have modified the original Pilates exercises, created by Joseph Pilates years ago, and updated them to suit our bodies' postural challenges in today's world. Therefore, it is very important that you read this chapter and assess your own posture to find out where you are tight, weak and have potential for long-term injury. If you currently have any kind of neck or back pain, this chapter is also critical for you to assess your possible issues. Without a thorough read of this section, it will be difficult to choose from the exercises in Chapter 8. The book is designed to not only teach you Pilates, but to teach you the best Pilates routine to help improve the shape of *your* body.

Chapter 3 on nutrition is a must-read for those looking to lose weight. Without proper food intake, the body will not drop the kilos. Your waist will not get smaller and your thighs will remain jiggly. Food intake is a crucial element to changing the way you look; therefore, we decided to write an entire chapter on it. We teach you *when* to eat, *what* to eat and *how* to eat. If your goal is to look like Katrina Kaif, then you must read Chapter 3.

Chapters 4 and 5 spend time on how to sit, stand, walk and breathe. These may seem irrelevant to looking fit, but you are wrong. You can spend 30 minutes a day exercising, but if you don't pay attention to your body the other 23.5 hours of the day, you can undo everything good about your workout. Without proper breathing, the abdominals cannot engage properly, making them look puffier than they really are. Improper everyday movement patterns such as incorrect sitting, standing and walking make you look slouchier, less energetic and, overall, less appealing.

Chapter 6 talks about fear. What does fear have to do with getting fit? Fear is the reason people lose motivation and it often determines whether we succeed or fail at achieving a goal. 'Well, I'm not scared of Pilates,' you say, and therefore skip this chapter . . . right? Well, we argue that the reason you picked up this book in the first place was because you really wanted to get into better shape. If it was that easy to have a perfect body, wouldn't you already have one? We encourage you to read this chapter and find out what deeply entrenched fears might be stopping you from having the body of your dreams. You may be surprised to find out something about yourself you never knew before.

Chapter 7 delves into how fitness can affect your emotions. Both authors of this book became fitness professionals not only to achieve great physiques, but also because of the way being fit made them feel. How you hold yourself in alignment can affect not only how you feel about yourself, but also how you are perceived by others. This chapter will also help you to achieve the important mind–body connection.

Chapter 8 finally delves into twenty-four hand-selected Pilates exercises that you can morph into a personalized workout. Each exercise is equipped with descriptions, modifications and advancements. There are pictures and cues to help you along the way. We recommend you find the exercises suited for your body and spend some time getting to know them. Do them one at a time, reading the descriptions and trying them out.

Chapter 9 is where you will learn how to 'change it up' for variety and how to make your workout flow better. It gives you sample workouts to change the order of the exercises, and gives you ideas on how to make it more challenging once you have been doing them for a while. We've also included five new abdominal exercises in this chapter for the ambitious exercisers who are looking for an additional challenge.

From beginning to end, we hope you enjoy the reading journey as much as we have enjoyed sharing it with you.

Turn the page, and let the learning begin!

WHAT IS PILATES?

Physical fitness is the first requisite of happiness.
Joseph Pilates, *Return to Life through Contrology*

You've picked up this book for a reason, and you are ready to get into the best shape of your life. You're ready for a flat stomach, firm arms, shapely legs and an amazing posture, right? Well, before we share all the secrets on how to achieve this, let's ask you a few questions:

When you rolled out of bed this morning, did your back and neck feel amazing and pain-free?

Are you able to climb two flights of stairs without stopping, or huffing and puffing at the top?

Do you look in the mirror and smile because your abdominals look as toned as Deepika Padukone's?

If handed a pair of running shoes, could you run a kilometre in under six minutes?

Could you pick up your six-year-old son, niece or grandson without fear of throwing your back out?

Do you eat your veggies at least three times a day?

Do you get on the scale every day and marvel at your perfect weight?

Is water the first thing you grab before any other beverage?

Do you flex your biceps and think, 'Yup, just like Hrithik's'?

If you answered 'yes' to all of these questions, you clearly have your health at the top of the priority list and you're at the top of your game.

For the rest of us, this is a wake-up call. It is possible to answer 'yes' to all of these questions. In this book you will learn that through proper exercise, you can considerably reduce your neck and back pain. Climbing stairs and running become easy with a regular routine, and picking up heavy children is a piece of cake when you're a Pilates enthusiast. You can look in the mirror someday and marvel at how your stomach is as flat as Malaika Arora Khan's. You can train yourself to eat vegetables, and you will learn that proper water consumption is the key to keeping all your body parts properly tuned.

Everything we quizzed you on above was taught to us by the man who created our own personal road map to health: Joseph Pilates. He created a methodology that teaches you to exercise in a way that guarantees higher endurance levels, better sleep and a calmer state of mind. Flat abs and toned, lean muscles are also a solid by-product of following the Pilates principles. It truly strengthens you from the inside out, and everything in between.

Can Pilates Help You Lose Weight?

This is one of the first questions we receive from every client looking to embark on a Pilates routine. Of course, Pilates helps you lose weight! But remember, Pilates is a long-term solution

(*Cont.*)

to weight loss and is definitely not your quick fix. One of the benefits of Pilates is that it builds muscle in the body. Each pound of muscle that we add to the body burns six times more calories than its fat counterpart. Therefore, adding muscle is key to increasing your metabolism and jump-starting the weight loss. In addition, Pilates muscles come from performing body weight exercises. If you are using the Pilates equipment, the weight that is loaded onto the muscle is very light. Therefore, you are not building significant amounts of mass. In most cases, lifting heavy weights with limited repetitions is the way to build a greater amount of muscle mass. Pilates does not take this approach. Everyone is different with regard to how their bodies react to stimuli and the kind of challenge it gives the muscles, but for most people, Pilates will give them a sleek and toned look, without making them excessively bulky. If you add proper diet into the mix, then losing weight will be heightened and quickened.

First, How Is Pilates Pronounced?

It is 'pilots' with an 'a', right? Not exactly.

Phonetically, it is spelled Pill-a-tees.

Pilates is the last name of the revolutionary man who brought us a system of exercises that can shape what we look like and who we are. We say 'who we are' because Pilates is not just a combination of movements; it's a philosophy. Joseph Pilates used exercise to fix everything, from your posture to your breathing to your immune system. He wanted you to be strong, powerful and happy.

Joseph Pilates died in the 1960s and his teachings did not gain much popularity until the late 1990s. It's a phenomenon now that has widespread appeal and has spawned a variety of different Pilates-like methodologies. Some compare Pilates to yoga, which is a confusion that is quite understandable. Like Pilates, yoga is a practice that involves more than just movement. There is breathing, there is mindfulness and there is a focus on the mind–body connection that is paramount to both practices. However, a majority of the exercises, the body positions, the pace and the flow, are different. While yoga emphasizes stretching and elongation of every element of the body, Pilates has a more strength-based approach. Pilates addresses a person's flexibility on a more practical and functional level. Either way, Pilates is a worldwide phenomenon, the popularity of which is fast approaching that of yoga, and is here to stay in our fitness world.

The age of sitting all the time—whether it is while we drive or while we work—has manufactured new aches and pains. Our shoulders are more rounded forward and our lower backs have lost their natural curve. We breathe differently because we are sitting on a chair all day. When you perform manual labour, you use your back muscles to pick up heavy objects and pull them around. With a sitting job, you use your wrists, fingers, neck and shoulders to do all the work. And mobile phones take postural issues to a whole new level. Looking down, using your hands and rounding forward for hours on end are sure to make you hunchbacked. People with a hunchback also often have a paunch as the result of a weak centre.

Doing Pilates regularly can fix all of these issues. It can give you a new posture, and reformed breathing and alignment. It can increase your energy. It can make you look taller. Most of all, you will feel better with a regular Pilates practice.

Who Was Joseph Pilates?

Here is your quick history lesson on Pilates. Don't skip it because it's important! Joseph Pilates was born in 1883 in Germany, to a father who was a gymnast and a mother who was a naturopath. It is said that his parents' passions influenced his upbringing and his eventual life-changing inventions.

Joseph Pilates was quite sick as a child, suffering from rickets and asthma, and his illnesses motivated him to pursue good health through physical activity. By the time he was fourteen years old, he had indulged in physical activities such as yoga, t'ai chi and bodybuilding, just to name a few. Over the years, he worked as a boxer and taught self-defence. He sculpted his body to such an extent that he was asked to pose for anatomical posters.

During World War I, Joseph moved to England. Since he was a German national, he was forced to enter an internment camp. His history of personal sickness motivated him to help others and get them into top physical condition. It was a day and age when there was not much for the sickly to do besides continue to be bedridden and get sicker. Joseph took it upon himself to teach people that physical exercise could help fight off disease. It was in the internment camp that he really started to expand the teachings of his exercise regimen. Since he grew tired of manually moving his patient's bodies, he pulled the springs off the beds to create assistance for his exercises. This was how the Pilates equipment was born.

Visualize this: sick patients in beds and wheelchairs using bed springs to perform exercises to heal themselves. Bed springs! There is a Pilates legend that says he trained over

8000 internees, of which none contracted influenza during the epidemic of 1918. Today, you would pop a decongestant and get back to work, but back then, there were no such options. Uncle Joe, as he was called, created a way. He became quite well known and loved as a nurse and physiotherapist, and was always inventing new ways to help both the doctors and the patients.

It was this vision of using bed springs to create resistance and build strength that led to the creation of his first piece of equipment, called the trapeze table (often also called the Cadillac—presumably due to the fact that it is a rather fine piece of equipment). The trapeze table still enjoys considerable popularity today due to its usability for any client at any level. Those with balance issues, or those with back pain, may enjoy the stability of a surface that does not move, and allows you to lie still while bringing the springs to you.

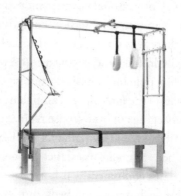

A Trapeze Table

Photo courtesy Balanced Body®

After World War I, Joseph returned to Germany and started training the Hamburg military police in self-defence. He was also asked to start working with the new German army, but his dislike for the direction that German politics was headed towards motivated him to leave the country.

In 1926, Joseph immigrated to the United States, landing in New York City. On the boat journey, he met his future life partner, Clara, who eventually became a long-term supporter of the exercise regime he called Contrology. He met Clara when she was suffering from arthritis, and Joseph helped her overcome this.

In New York, he opened his studio at 939 Eighth Avenue, in a gymnasium adjacent to many dance studios. For this reason, many people mistakenly assume that he was a dancer. In time, word simply spread of his ability to heal bodies and create significant strength in the muscles needed to create intricate movements. Huge names in the dance community like Martha Graham and George Balanchine would go to Joseph to get 'fixed'. Joseph wrote numerous books, the most well known of which was *Return to Life*, and he continued to invent equipment and develop his methodology well into his eighties. He died in 1967 of emphysema.

Clara continued Joseph's work for ten years after his death, and a group of instructors, commonly called the Pilates Elders, also spread his method around the world. One of the elders, named Ron Fletcher, was among the first to bring Pilates to Beverly Hills, where the celebrities began to practise it. In 1972, the Ron Fletcher Studio for Body Contrology opened up on Rodeo Drive in Beverly Hills, and attracted the likes of Barbra Streisand, Candice Bergen and Nancy Reagan.

Wasn't Pilates a Dancer?

Pilates is usually performed with pointed toes, graceful arms and rhythmic movement. I (Zeena) was introduced to Pilates for the first time ever when I was nineteen years old, in a dance class in college. We did this thing called the hundreds (featured in Chapter 9) and huffed and puffed our way through a bunch of difficult core exercises. I figured, back then, that this was just another kind of dance workout, created by some crazy, strong dancer who wanted us to work from our centre. But Joseph Pilates himself was not a dancer. Uncle Joe had set up shop in a gymnasium in NYC, in the same building where many famous dancers rehearsed. This proximity to the community, combined with Joseph's slow, graceful movements, made it easy for dancers to embrace his work. To this day, a majority of instructors pursuing Pilates as a career in the US come from a movement- and dance-based background. It's a wonderful way to mix what you love (movement), with helping people change how they look and feel.

It's clear that Joseph Pilates was ahead of his time. Twenty years after his death, what he had started began to gain widespread popularity. In the early 2000s, Pilates exploded and began to cross time zones to become an international phenomenon.

In India, the popularity of Pilates is still in its infancy. When I (Yasmin) travelled to the US to receive my certification in the Pilates method in 2006, I was one of the first Indians to do so and get full training. My studio, Body Image, was the first in Mumbai to offer actual equipment-based training, and I have become one of the very few top-notch Pilates instructors in India. In fact, when the time came to purchase equipment for my studio from the manufacturers in the US, the customs fees to get the equipment to India cost as much as the equipment itself! I travelled home from my first trip to California, stuffing my suitcase with as many Pilates props as possible, barely leaving room for anything else.

Learning Pilates

When I (Yasmin) first made inquiries with regard to taking my Pilates certification in the States, I was told I needed to have prior experience with Pilates. How was I going to get Pilates experience if I was the first to really teach Pilates in my country? I convinced them that I was experienced (having then been in the fitness industry for twelve years), got them to understand my predicament and arrived for my course filled with confidence and excitement. I then found myself incredibly intimidated by the myriad dancers and physical therapists in my course. The dancers were very coordinated, rhythmic and knew how to let the movements flow as required in Pilates. The physical therapists were filled with knowledge and education beyond my own. However, I found my strengths. I practised and practised until I felt the movement deep inside my body. I didn't let intimidation rule my desires, and went on to pass my course with flying colours.

We estimate that the percentage of clients doing Pilates in India likely resembles the percentage of people doing Pilates in the US ten to fifteen years ago. Gyms still do not offer it, and clients still remain confused about the difference between

Pilates and its counterpart, yoga. We venture to guess that the explosion is still to come. We believe that the desire of Indians across the country to feel stronger in their core, stand taller, feel leaner and improve their posture will continue to grow. Pilates can offer this, and so much more, to our population. We hope that more studios will pop up around the country and educate people about the power of this exercise methodology.

The word 'Pilates' is used everywhere now, due to a failed trademark lawsuit in a Manhattan federal court (in the year 2000) which gave the rights of the word to everyone. A lot of what is being taught as Pilates bears little resemblance to the original repertoire that Joseph created. As we have embraced the principles created by him, we feel confident that he would embrace the changes that have been incorporated, as long as those changes come with strong reasoning. Joseph had a powerful, inventive mind, and we believe that the changes to his methodology proposed in the very book you are reading would have been blessed by Joseph himself.

What we call Pilates (and often struggle to pronounce correctly) was called Contrology by Joseph himself. The word 'control' offers significant perspective on what he was trying to accomplish. Do you feel like you often have no control over your life and your body? With Contrology, you can reverse that. Instead of floating through exercises without thinking about them, you move with intention, with purpose and with control. Joseph's exercises were meant to address a myriad of problems. He wanted to build strong muscles and an ideal posture.

In his book, Joseph addresses a lot of physical, mental and spiritual issues. In addition to outlining the specifics of each of his 34 prescribed exercises, he advises on how to sleep, eat, breathe and bathe. Yes, we said 'bathe'. He suggests using a good 'stiff brush' to scrub every portion of your body and he even encourages you to 'contort' into positions to get yourself clean. He discusses breathing, and how it contributes to circulation of the blood. He urges you not to eat in excess, and advises you to sleep within a ventilated room and on a firm mattress. He encourages you to 'never slouch', but not for obvious reasons, like preventing neck and back pain. He makes the link between poor posture and the compression of the lungs and vital organs. He argues that once your body is in great condition, your mind and your spirit will be able to handle the demands of modern culture. Even in 1947, he was able to see the detrimental effects that civilized society had on our long-term health and longevity.

Joseph Pilates also spent time addressing our aversion to exercises and propensity towards laziness. He advised his readers not to give into temptation and take a night off from their routine. He calls this a 'momentary weakness', and advises you to remain 'true to yourself'. He was a living example of his work, practising his principles and exercise well into his eighties. Reading Joseph's book *Return to Life* is like reading the notes of your loving, strict, compassionate and strong-willed grandfather.

To say the authors of this book are devotees of his work is an understatement. We may change his choreography, and we may adjust the order of exercises. We may have differing opinions on what's appropriate for today's bodies and lives, but one fact remains the same: we believe in the power of a strong mind and a strong body. By reading this book and following the guidelines we lay out for you, we are simply allowing the inspiration of one man to transcend time and distance. He claimed that his word was fifty years ahead of his time. More than fifty years later, we are still inspired.

The Six Principles of Pilates

There are six main principles of Pilates: concentration, control, centre, flow, precision and breath. It is important to know and understand these principles. You will see them in every exercise we teach.

Concentration: The ability to focus on what you are doing, as you are doing it. No chit-chat, no mind chatter, no singing along with your music while you do your exercises. Concentrate. On. Each. Movement. Did your mind wander just now? Bring it back, and concentrate.

Control: This is the essence of the original work, and is something we aim for in every movement. You may move fast, you may move slowly, but move always with control. In equipment Pilates (Reformer, Cadillac, Wunda Chair), one of our favourite sentences, which we keep repeating to our clients, is: 'Don't let the spring control you; you are in control of the spring.' Only you can create this control within your own body.

Centre: This is where movement begins and ends. It's deep within your abdominals. It includes your butt muscles, inner thighs and back muscles. Without a strong centre, the movement is superficial. Do you feel like you have a layer of fat over this centre? Continue reading to learn how to get stronger and get rid of this belly fat so that you can truly find your centre.

Flow: Have you ever wanted to move like a dancer? Walk the runway like a model? This principle of flow is essential in teaching you how to move gracefully and efficiently. Movements should not be sharp and jerky. They should flow smoothly, and your routine should make you feel like you are floating on water. Once control and concentration are mastered, flow will naturally take its course. When you flow through each movement without stopping, maximum stamina and endurance are developed.

Precision: Arguably one of the more important principles, precision is something we pride ourselves on as Pilates practitioners. In our teaching, you will come across instructions like, 'The head cannot tilt forward in this exercise, since it strains the cervical spine,' or, 'Yes, the knees should be together to maximize glute activation.' These are just two examples of how precise we are in our teaching, and how important precision can be to movement. Pilates is based on a foundation of precise movements. Know where your foot is, where your hand is, and even where your fingers are placed. Each detail has a precise purpose.

Breath: An entire chapter of this book is dedicated to breath and its importance in Pilates. One of the first things to learn when practising Pilates is how to breathe in and out without letting go of the abdominal muscles. In Pilates we learn to breathe into the ribcage, we breathe in through the nose, we breathe out through the mouth, and we relax our neck and shoulders. But more importantly, with every movement, we breathe. Because without breath, there is no powerful life.

Types of Pilates

We are frequently asked, 'What is the difference between mat Pilates and equipment Pilates?' Pricing aside (equipment Pilates will usually be more expensive), both practices utilize the six principles stated above.

Mat Pilates: Joseph Pilates created 34 exercises that are performed on the mat in a certain sequence. All that is needed is the mat, your body and your six principles. If you are practising classical Pilates, or the exercises described in the exact order and repetition as laid out by Joseph himself years ago, you will do a mat class exactly the same every time. However, in today's society, instructors and studios practise a more contemporary style, which means that they have modified the original exercises to suit their own style of teaching. The exercises may be different and performed in a different order. This book emphasizes a contemporary style of Pilates, and will actually allow you to 'choose your own adventure' for the exercises you want to do. Mat Pilates excels in its convenience and accessibility to all. You can perform mat Pilates anywhere and any time, and many students can be packed into a mat Pilates class, making the price lower and the class more accessible to all.

Equipment Pilates: There are twenty inventions that Pilates patented over the years. The most popular of these machines is the universal Reformer, which is a bed-like apparatus with a moveable carriage and straps for the hands and feet. This machine is the most popular one in the market and has inspired various versions, from higher Reformers to assist those in physical therapy, to inexpensive, floor-based models made for home use.

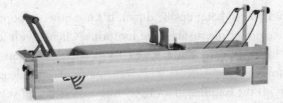

A Reformer

Photo courtesy Balanced Body®

What is that equipment?

When I (Zeena) encountered Pilates for the second time, it was still in its infancy in the US. I was getting married and looking for a way to sculpt my abs in time to wear my stomach-exposing lehenga. I drove by a small studio with four machines butted up against each other and barely any room to move. This was Pilates? I thought it was only done on the mat. My super-fit male instructor put me on a Reformer for the first time and I was intimidated. It looked like a torture device! All the pulleys, springs, settings and bars made my head spin. He was a skilled instructor who knew just what to say and how to keep me motivated. What I found was that I could feel my muscles better, and hit positions that I could barely hit on the mat. My back felt amazing after the workout and I was covered in perspiration. I left the studio quivering; I was hooked on this Reformer thing, and had to learn more.

The Trapeze Table (or, as Joseph called it, the 'Cadillac' of all machines) is a higher table with poles and straps. This machine boasts of easy-to-manipulate springs and poles, and allows you to hang upside down. It's not quite as popular as the Reformer due to its large footprint. Clients with injuries will love using the Cadillac due to its wide surface area and unmoving table. Clients who want more of a challenge will hang off the Cadillac in a variety of positions to allow gravity to provide resistance to the core.

Another machine called the Wunda Chair (named thus because it can do wonders for you) actually also functioned as a piece of furniture in Joseph's apartment. This is proof of how he lived and breathed his work. Joseph claimed, 'It will give you the surprise of your life and make you "Wunda" when you witness an exhibition covering more than 100 different exercises.' The Wunda Chair is much smaller and more portable than the other two machines. With this smaller surface area and footprint, come significantly more challenges to stability and balance.

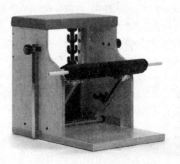

A Wunda Chair

Photo courtesy Balanced Body®

Joseph was a constant inventor and innovator, and often used everyday items to help him create the equipment he needed to do his work. For example, apparently his ladder barrel was first created from a beer keg. It's also claimed that he used the rings from a beer keg to create his first Magic Circle—another piece of equipment.

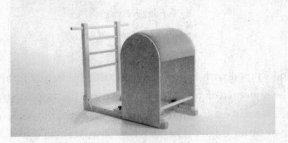

A Ladder Barrel

Photo courtesy Balanced Body®

The most beneficial aspect of Pilates equipment is its ability to either assist a client with a movement, or add challenge to a movement. There are a significantly higher number of exercises that can be performed, in a variety of different positions. We can stand, sit, lie down, lie sideways, or either hang upside down or with the right side up, all on the Pilates equipment. Usually, equipment work is done in much smaller groups, so that the attention to detail and precision will be paramount. Of course, this makes the pricing of equipment sessions much higher and not as accessible to all clients.

Pilates with props: There are numerous small props that can be used to assist in the Pilates workout, both on the equipment and on the mat. The most recognizable is the Pilates Ring, or Magic Circle.

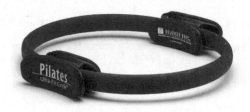

A Pilates Ring

Photo courtesy Balanced Body®

Round shaped with a strong but flexible framework, the ring can be squeezed if pressure is placed on the opposing hand pads. This can create muscle load on the arms, the core, or the inner or outer thighs. The Fletcher Towel is also a wonderful tool that helps clients engage their scapula muscles, which are important for postural training. Thera-Bands give more resistance and can be used for hamstring stretching and simple arm work. Small balls are placed under the tail bone or between the inner thighs to challenge the body in a new way. Bigger balls can be added to the workout to increase a balance challenge. Our favourite balance tool, the BOSU Ball, is wonderful because its half-dome offers the client the ability to perform an entire abdominal sequence on the bouncy, unstable surface.

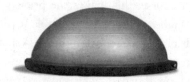

Bosu Ball

Classical Pilates: Whether it's performed on the mat or with the equipment, classical mat Pilates refers to the Pilates exercises as they were created by Joseph many years ago. Classical enthusiasts usually prefer the mat classes to be taught in the same particular order that Joseph originally intended them to be in. Classical work also involves a great deal of 'round-back' exercises, meaning that the lower back and spine tend to be rounded (refer to page 119: 'Rolling Like a Ball'). This feels wonderful for clients with healthy spines, and can help create length and flexibility in the muscles around the vertebrae. However, many clients come to Pilates instructors already experiencing back pain, and this classical position can sometimes be contraindicated for their particular injury. Clients with osteoporosis must also avoid this position.

Contemporary Pilates: Again, whether performed on equipment or the mat, contemporary Pilates refers to the way the exercises are taught. The order, the body position and the pace can all determine whether a class is classical or contemporary. Most of what is being offered in India follows the contemporary style. Both authors of this book teach contemporary Pilates, and what you will read in the coming pages is very contemporary. We have taken the original work created by Joseph years ago, and changed the body position. We also teach classes outside the original order. It is the belief of instructors who teach a contemporary style that Pilates himself would have encouraged us to make changes to his original work. These changes reflect the changes in our culture, our postures, our spines, our chronic injuries and our lifestyle. We still teach many exercises in the 'round-back' position, however, there is less emphasis on this and there is more emphasis on the neutral lower-back position.

Regardless of whether the preference is equipment or mat, why do we practise and encourage contemporary Pilates? Why not follow exactly what Joseph laid out for us almost ninety years ago?

Well, let's look at what was going on in the world when Joseph was alive and kicking in New York City. It was the roaring twenties. People drove cars, but not nearly as far or as long as we do today. There were no computers in sight, no mobile phones in every hand and no call centres where people sit for hours on end. People walked around town and carried their purchases. Manual labour was the most common way to earn wages. They sat upright on horses and elephants and rode around town. Their posture was different. So, how do we evolve with the changing times? We make the original work contemporary, to suit our changing lifestyle. As we mentioned before, we believe that if Joseph were alive today, he would embrace a new vision of how to fix our bodies.

Pilates as an industry is constantly evolving. Large manufacturers of fitness equipment are taking Joseph's idea of using bed springs for assistance and resistance, and creating new innovations every year. Wunda Chairs now have pedals that are split for each leg. They can be stacked, and easily lifted and moved. Reformers now come with 'towers' attached that can mimic the exercise done on a Cadillac, in a much smaller machine. Foam Rollers now have springs attached to add arm work and leg work. One of the largest manufacturers of Pilates equipment has produced a new upright machine called CoreAlign® which brings the principles of Pilates into a standing, upright position.

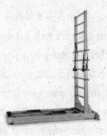

CoreAlign

Photo courtesy Balanced Body®

Many forms of exercise have spawned from the original Pilates repertoire and taken on a life of their own. Some gyms have combined the yoga and Pilates elements together for fusion classes such as 'piyo' and 'yogilates'. The Barre Method is probably the most popular and fastest-growing segment of the Pilates spin-off market. Barre combines ballet movements with Pilates to create a low-cost, mat-based workout that involves a lot of standing positions. Another equipment-based Pilates spin-off is the Megaformer, created by Hollywood celebrity trainer Sebastien Lagree. Much like a regular Reformer, the Megaformer uses springs and straps to create a resistance-based workout. The list of Pilates-based workouts goes on, and as the years go by, many new ones will arrive and fade.

Sophie Choudry on training with the latest equipment

As a kid back in London, I used to see my mum's passion for Pilates. In fact, she sent me for my first class when I was just sixteen. I did Pilates for a while but it was only years later, in Mumbai, that I developed a true passion for it. Fitness has always been an important part of my lifestyle. However, a couple of years ago, I suffered from a slipped disc in my neck and, a year later, one in my lower back. That was the end of my weight training and yoga for a while. What saved me was Pilates with Yasmin Karachiwala, so much so that I was able to take part in the extremely physically challenging Jhalak Dikhla Jaa *stunts. I never thought I would! The best part about training with Yasmin is that she constantly updates herself with all the latest techniques and machines. Be it CoreAlign®, Reformer, Cadillac or Core Barre, each piece of equipment pushes you to challenge yourself.*

Why Choose Contemporary Pilates?

Joseph Pilates's original work consisted of multiple exercises in a position we call spinal flexion. There are a few kinds of spinal flexion, and they are dependent on what part of your back is actually flexed. In some cases, this is thoracic flexion, which makes up the middle twelve vertebrae of your spine:

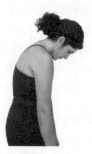

Thoracic Flexion

Often, flexion also includes lumbar flexion which involve the lower five vertebrae of your spine.

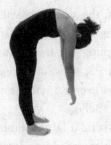

Lumbar Flexion

In both cases, these positions usually require cervical flexion, which includes the top seven vertebrae.

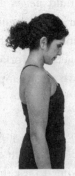

Cervical Flexion

These exercises work the superficial abdominal muscles, such as the rectus abdominis, very well. You will feel the burn in your stomach after holding this position for ten seconds or longer. Once your body starts to fatigue in this position, your neck muscles will get tired and you may start to feel strained. In addition, the shoulders will round forward into the hunchback sitting position we described, which people who sit at the computer for long hours suffer from. Sure, doing this exercise made sense in the early 1900s but today, for most people, this exercise will simply strain their necks and make their backs ache.

Why should we spend a large amount of time during our Pilates routine in this rounded position when we are already so rounded? We are working abdominal muscles, but there are actually a number of lesser-known and lesser-performed Pilates exercises that work these abdominals, open up the posture, and provide what we need to build a strong centre. We're not saying you should *never* do the 'hundreds'; we are merely reminding you to be cognizant of your posture and your exercise selection. You will learn in Chapter 8 that it is very possible to get the workout you want without emphasizing this posture we are attempting to avoid.

What Is NOT Pilates?

Any uneducated consumer can argue that every abs-strengthening exercise we do can be called Pilates. Since it became acceptable for anyone to use the term 'Pilates', often, the work gets muddled and confused. We have our answers:

We believe doing 100 crunches a day is *not* Pilates.

We affirm that mindless chatting in class while swinging your legs around in circles is *not* Pilates.

We passionately believe that pushing yourself so hard that you can't walk the next day from soreness is *not* Pilates.

We guarantee that anything that hurts your back and strains your muscles is *not* Pilates.

Pilates Precautions

We will talk more in Chapter 8 about specific exercises to avoid for certain demographics; however, overall, Pilates is pretty safe for the general public. With slow, controlled movements and attention to precision, Pilates is far less likely to hurt you than, say, a kick-boxing class or boot camp. However, if you have a diagnosed spinal condition such as spinal stenosis or spinal spondylosis, it is highly recommended that you get permission and guidelines from your doctor with regard to what your body can handle. People with osteoporosis in the hips or spine should also be careful not to do too much flexion (bending forward) of the spine. This book eliminates a lot of the excessive flexion and, therefore, can be appropriate for the osteoporosis client. However, it is still important to proceed with caution and get your doctor's permission.

Pregnant clients cannot spend excessive amounts of time on their back after the first trimester; therefore, they too will have to remove a significant number of exercises from the Pilates mat repertoire. Equipment Pilates, with its ability to modify exercises, is far better suited to the pregnant client. Overall, Pilates in some form can be practised by nearly everyone, but taking precautions is always a smart choice when beginning a new exercise routine.

Coming Up Next

Now you know a bit about Joseph Pilates: where he came from, how his work evolved and what makes it different from other workouts. You should also have a good understanding of why we are suggesting some changes in the original Pilates repertories in order to accommodate our changing bodies and lifestyles. In the next chapter, we will spend some time teaching you about your posture and how it could be morphing into something that is causing you pain and making you look bigger and sloppier than you really are. You will learn how to assess your own posture so that when the time comes to create your own Pilates workout, you can make an educated selection of exercises to perform daily. With concentration, control and precision, we will provide you with the tools that Pilates originally intended, to help you look and feel better. We will do this without creating bigger postural problems; instead, we will help you to counteract the demands of life in today's world. This revolutionary methodology created years ago promises to help you 'return to life'.

As Joseph said in his *Return to Life through Contrology*, 'Contrology develops the body uniformly, corrects wrong postures, restores physical vitality, invigorates the mind, and elevates the spirit.'

SHAPING GOOD POSTURE

*Good posture can be successfully acquired only when the
entire mechanism of the body is under perfect control*
        Joseph Pilates, *Return to Life through Contrology*

One of the first things that we look at as instructors is the
'shape' of a client's body. In reality, we are referring to their
posture. Posture is a very powerful tool to help you look and
feel better. It's at the core of this book and is the key to how
you will design you own Pilates workout.

The word 'posture' is very powerful. It acts as both a noun
and a verb. As a noun, it is used thus: 'I love your standing
posture.' As a verb: 'She is posturing for her position as the
leader.' With regard to this book, both definitions of the word
imply one thing: that the position of individual body parts is
of paramount importance to the overall effect of the sum of
the body parts put together.

When you use the word 'posture' as a noun, it is related
to the body. When used as a verb, it implies that you are
aligning yourself with a particular mindset. We love both
uses of this powerful word. The body needs to be aligned,
and if your mind is in alignment with it, it can result in
an extremely powerful and dynamic you. You will look

leaner. You will stand taller. You will be a commanding presence.

So, do you want to be seen as successful, lean and powerful? Posture is your answer. Take a look around the next time you are out and about. Who catches your eye? Is it the tall man in the sharp suit? Take a closer look. Maybe it's his posture that caught your attention. Now see if you can find an older person with a hunchback. What does this say to you? Perhaps all you see is how old he is and how he can't walk or move quickly. Now take a look at a teenager on a cellphone. Most likely, he is hunched over it and texting away. Does this even catch your attention? Probably not.

> Did you know that good posture increases energy? When your ribcage is in the correct position, you can take in more air. The more oxygen you breathe, the more energy you have.

In terms of body positioning, a good posture is key to long-term injury prevention. Our muscles hold our joints in alignment so that they may move efficiently and effectively. However, if the muscles get tight and weak, which is what happens when your posture is imperfect, the joints also move out of alignment. Soon the knee aches, the shoulder pinches and the hip begins to click. Instead of treating the pain, which is only a symptom, how about looking at the cause? In a lot of cases, improper postural alignment is the cause.

Did you know that correct posture decreases your chances of neck and back pain? The more aligned your spine is, the less your back and neck muscles become strained or overworked.

In the following pages, we will discuss the various elements of posture. Firstly, what are the proper body mechanics needed to place your bones in proper alignment? Secondly, how does good or bad posture affect your attitude and how people see you? You will also learn how your poor posture is making you look bigger, fatter, wider and far less appealing.

There are three major postural misalignments we plan to focus on. We will describe them in depth and teach you how to assess your postural problem area. Once you complete your self-assessments, you will be guided through the Pilates exercises best suited to your needs.

Did you know that postural-alignment exercises can improve other joint-related ailments of the knees, hips and ankles? When the pelvis is in the incorrect position, certain muscles don't work well, placing undue stress on the lower limb joints.

A study published in the *International Journal of Scientific and Technology Research* in 2013 that tracked 400 IT professionals in India, stated that 51 per cent of the participants reported lower back pain, and that this was the number one musculoskeletal disorder of employees in that industry. Unless the pain is caused by some sort of impact injury, we know these issues are a result of poor posture. If our spine is not aligned properly because of sitting or driving all day long, the muscles don't function properly and get tight and sore.

Why Does Back Pain Get Worse as We Age?

Our chronic misalignments get worse over time from years of repetitive actions. When we are children, things are usually in place. We haven't yet sat at a desk, driven a car, bent over a phone or stood hunched in a kitchen for hours on end. We are playing, jumping, lifting things and sleeping. Therefore, children are often immune to postural alignment injuries. How many kids do you know under the age of ten who need to see a chiropractor?

Did you know that correcting your posture can reduce your chances of carpel tunnel symptoms (pain in the hands and fingers, which can arise as a result of excessive texting and computer work)? When the cervical spine (neck area) is out of alignment, it can negatively impact how you hold your shoulders, elbows and wrists. When the tendons in the wrist get strained, pain can radiate into the hands.

In our years of teaching precise and specific Pilates movements, we have successfully helped people to eliminate back pain, neck pain, jaw pain, headaches and migraines. 'How?' you ask. Based on the simple idea of placing the parts of the body back where they are supposed to be.

Visualize a set of building blocks stacked on top of each other. If each part of each square is not exactly aligned with the others, how stable is your structure? If something is misaligned and out of place, does the centre line of the structure still have its integrity? The answer is 'no', and your body works the same way.

Did you know that improving your posture can add more muscle definition and contribute to a leaner appearance? Great back muscles and glutes (butt muscles) are a direct result of doing exercise in the proper postural position. If your pelvis is in the correct position, it can make your waist look smaller. If your spine is aligned, the back muscles will appear more defined.

In fact, the body is more intricate than a simple set of building blocks. The joints are supposed to be held together by the muscles. However, when the muscles get tight, weak or overused, the joints move further and further out of alignment, the result being poor posture.

Below you will see a picture illustrating proper posture. You will see a line drawn down through the midline of the body, starting from the ear, moving down into the shoulder, through the hips, the centre of the knee joint, and just in front of the ankle bones. This is called the 'plumb line'. Our goal is to get to this proper alignment, and most people have some sort of misalignment that deviates from this ideal.

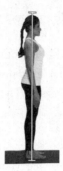

The plumb line may be straight up and down, but the spine is in an S shape with a few natural curves.

The degrees of these curves are limited, and when the curves become excessive due to poor posture and incorrect movement patterns, we have the 'postural misalignments' described below:

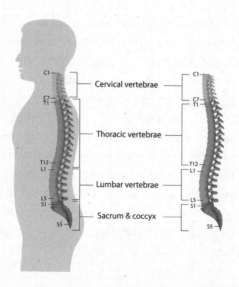

- The first seven top vertebrae of the spine are collectively called the 'cervical spine'. Imagine you are looking at yourself from the side. The C shape is facing backwards from the midline of the body.

- The next twelve vertebrae are called the 'thoracic spine'. The C shape is facing forward from the midline of the body towards the front of you.

- The bottom five vertebrae are called the 'lumbar spine'. The C shape is facing backwards from the midline of the body.

If the words 'cervical', 'thoracic' and 'lumbar' are too much for you to remember, we have just the trick to help you recall the order. Just think of your spine as a meal: the top is 'breakfast', the middle is 'lunch' and the bottom is 'dinner'. We provide cues to our clients by using these words occasionally, and we may include them in some of our other discussions. So if I tell you to keep your 'dinner' in check, it means you might be forgetting the proper position of your lumbar (lower) spine.

Below, we discuss three major postural deviations that are seen in the majority of the population. One of these postures—the hunchback—will describe what happens most often with the upper body, and the other two—arched back and flat back—will describe what can happen to the lower half.

Upper-Body Postural Deviations

Kyphosis, or Hunchback Posture

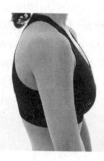

We believe this ails at least 90 per cent of the people reading this book. Unless you regularly engage in alignment-focused workouts, such as Pilates or yoga, chances are you have a hunchback posture.

The head is usually in front of the shoulders. Notice that the ends of the shoulders are facing forward, towards the front of the room, as opposed to the sides of the room. The C curve of the thoracic spine is more excessive than it should be. If you look from behind, it's often difficult to see the outline of the scapula, or the shoulder blades. Basically, your 'breakfast' and 'lunch' are out of alignment.

You will notice this posture in people with desk jobs, in the older population, in women with larger breast sizes, in teenagers who are glued to their cellphones and just about anyone else who doesn't pay attention to the problem. With the head weighing eight lbs or more (3.6 kg), this bowling ball, sitting on the front of the shoulder joint can eventually make the neck feel stiff and sore. The rounded shoulders can cause injury to the shoulder joint and rotator cuff.

Have you ever wondered why you see men lifting shoulder-weights and then rubbing their shoulders and shaking off the pain? We believe this comes from lifting heavy weights and doing so without the shoulder joint being in the right postural position. The poor joint is being asked to move with efficiency, without being stacked properly on its preceding block.

Have you ever wondered why your neck hurts from sitting at your desk for a while, and why neck massages only help for a few hours and, eventually, the pain returns? This comes from the constant pressure of the 'bowling ball' leaning forward in a position that is unnatural and unintended. The building blocks are off course, and the muscles around it were not meant to handle this load.

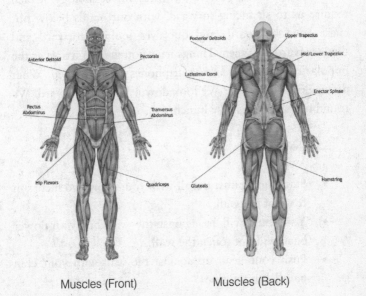

Muscles (Front)   Muscles (Back)

Hunchback-posture muscle features include:

   i.   Tight pectoral (chest) muscles
  ii.   Tight latissimus dorsi (sides of the back) muscles
 iii.   Tight upper trapezius (neck) muscles
 iv.   Weak erector spinae (around the spine) muscles
  v.   Weak mid/lower trapezius (mid-back) muscles
 vi.   Weak deep cervical spine (neck) muscles
vii.   Weak posterior deltoid (back of shoulders) muscles

This is the only upper-body postural misalignment we will address since it's the only one that runs rampant in today's hunched-over society. This particular issue has exacerbated over the years due to our advances in technology, which require us to sit facing forward, with our hands below our chest on a keyboard, and our eyes looking forward and down towards a screen. Things have gotten even worse as the popularity of texting and smartphones has exploded. What do we do all day long? We look down. We lean forward. We round our shoulders. We hunch.

ASSESSMENT:

- Stand up against a wall with your heels two inches in front of the wall.
- Your butt will be against the wall but your lower back will not touch the wall.
- Push your head up against the wall with your chin parallel to the floor.

- Make sure your front ribs are not sticking out and jutting forward. Pull your ribs into your spine.
- Are you able to feel the back of your shoulders against the wall? If not, you have a hunchback posture.
- If you feel your shoulders against the wall, does doing so require you to stick your ribs out and work really hard? If so, you have a hunchback posture.

Why Bother?

If fixing your posture to avoid long-term pain is not enough motivation for you, then let's look at how it affects your appearance. We all want to look lean and trim, correct? Well, for women with a hunchback posture, the breasts are going to sit much lower and closer to the waist, giving the illusion of a bigger midsection. The whole body shrinks, decreasing height and making you look shorter. Whether you have a flat stomach or not, the waist area is less defined since the fat in your whole midsection squishes together to form a thicker and more rounded appearance. Does that motivate you enough? The hunchback is a chronic postural problem that gets worse every year, especially for the younger and more technology-savvy generations.

Don't worry; you're reading the right book! Keep moving through the chapters and you will learn the correct Pilates-based exercises to align your shoulders, back and head, and decrease any neck pain you may be experiencing.

Lower-Body Postural Deviations

Lumbar Lordosis, or Arched-Back Posture

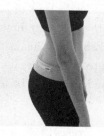

Arched back demonstration

Lordosis (arched back) is a very common problem, and usually occurs in conjunction with kyphosis (hunchback). This posture is often seen in clients who sit at a desk or at a computer all day long. The lower back arches excessively, causing a deeper C shape of the lumbar spine.

If you examine this posture, you can see how excessive jumping, lifting, running or even stretching, with the back in this position, can place pressure on the vertebra in the lumbar spine, causing compression, disc issues and lower back pain.

Arched-back-posture muscle features include:

i.   Tight hip flexor (front of the hips) muscles
ii. Tight erector spinae (sides of the spine) muscles
iii. Tight latissimus dorsi (sides of the back) muscles
iv. Weak deep intrinsic abdominal (stomach) muscles
v. Weak gluteus medius and maximus (butt) muscles

The goal of any exercise routine for someone with this posture is to bring the pelvis back into a more neutral position, where there is more of a natural C shape in the spine. This means finding exercises that emphasize stretching the hip flexors, strengthening the glutes and deepening the strength of the all-important abdominals. The core strengthening components of a regular Pilates practice can assist in correcting this postural misalignment.

Let's take a moment to talk about the abs. It is mentioned above that one set of muscles that needs to be strengthened, given this posture, are the abdominal muscles. However, if you look closely, you will see that it says the 'deep intrinsic abdominal' muscles. What does this mean, and what is the difference?

There is a multitude of muscles in the abdominal region—most obviously, the rectus abdominis (RA), the transversus abdominis (TVA) and the internal and external obliques. The RA refers to the muscles on the topmost layer, and these muscles are responsible for doing the 'crunching' action that we see in a lot of the Pilates exercises. Below the RA is the TVA, which wraps around the waist like a corset, and assists in stabilizing the pelvis. The obliques run diagonally on the sides of the abdominal region and are responsible for creating rotation and side movements of the spine.

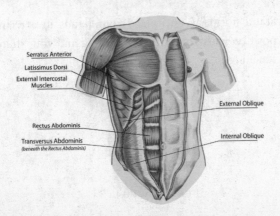

Serratus Anterior
Latissimus Dorsi
External Intercostal
Muscles

External Oblique

Rectus Abdominis

Internal Oblique

Transversus Abdominis
(beneath the Rectus Abdominis)

Most people want a flat, well-defined stomach, which means bulking up the RA muscle and shedding the fat on top of the muscle. However, it is the TVA that will really help to adjust the posture above, and create true strength in the inner muscles of the abdominal region. What does this mean when it comes to exercise selection? It means that excessive crunches, which predominantly utilize the RA, are not necessary. Excessive crunches are especially unnecessary when you perform these crunch-type exercises by rounding your upper spine forward and accentuating the hunchback posture.

You will notice as you get to the exercise-selection portion of the book, that we have primarily selected exercises that will still strengthen the abdominals without placing you in this forward-folding, crunched position. Trust us, exercises like 'front support' (see page 154) will get your belly feeling warm and worked. We will also provide exercises that will work your glutes and stretch the regions of your back that need to be elongated.

ASSESSMENT:

- Stand normally and place your hands in a triangle position with your fingers touching and your thumbs touching.

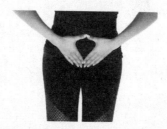

- Place this triangle on your stomach area, with your fingertips touching your pubic bone, and your thumbs below your belly button.
- Look down at your hand. Are your thumbs protruding forward more than your fingers? If so, then the top of your pelvis leans forward more, which means you have an arched-back posture.

A model testimonial

I (Yasmin) had a client who came to me after a successful year of walking the runway as a model. However, her career was threatened due to the intense back pain she was experiencing. Upon evaluating her body and posture, I determined right away that she had lordosis, or arched-back posture. This is quite common for models, since they tend to stick out their chests and butts in an attempt to look confident and shapely. However, without strong core muscles, this position can cause stress on the lower back. Luckily for this client, the solution was simple. Using Pilates as our tool, I strengthened her abdominals and stretched her hip flexors. We did many of the exercises in the 'arched back' section of this book (Chapter 8), in addition to exercises on the Reformer. Within weeks, she was in a condition to walk the runway and resume her career. What was the added bonus? The Pilates flattened her stomach and made her glutes more shapely.

Why Bother?

Let's look at how an arched-back posture can make you look less appealing and less slim. The booty (as we like to lovingly refer to it) sticks out further than it should, giving the appearance of a larger, less-toned butt. Even more tragic is the fact that the abdominals are weaker in this posture and tend to protrude as a result of the pelvis tipping forward. When the glutes and abs are in this position, it is harder to contract them and suck them in, as most people do when it's time to be on display. So just think—by simply getting your pelvis back where it needs to be, your abs and butt can look more toned and attractive. Lastly, any excess curvature of the spine will make you look shorter. Tall and lean is best achieved with perfect alignment.

Posterior Pelvic Posture, or Flat-Back Posture

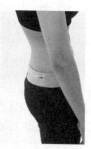

Flatback demonstration

Have you ever wondered why you've been unable to achieve a nice, rounded butt, and instead, your behind looks flat and wide? This could be because you have flat-back posture, also referred to as a posterior pelvic tilt. With this posture, the lumbar spine has little or no C curve. This posture is less common, but equally dangerous to the spine as we age. Walking becomes more difficult since the glutes are non-existent, and knee issues are often a problem with this posture since these glutes can't keep the knees in proper alignment with the toes. Much like those with an arched back, people with flat backs also have a hunchback posture, which, in turn, makes it look like the whole body is rounding forward into a big large C in the wrong direction.

Flat-back-posture muscle features include:

  i.   Tight hamstring (back of thigh) muscles
 ii.   Tight abdominal (centre) muscles
iii.   Weak gluteus (butt) muscles
 iv.   Weak hip flexors (front of hip)

Once again, you can see how targeted Pilates exercises can combat the flat-butt posture, and help give you great function in your spine (and a nice-looking behind). You will see in this posture that the abdominals are tight. Do you think doing excessive crunches with this posture would be a good thing? No, it wouldn't! We will find ways to work the core, but help release the tightness in the midsection and get the pelvis back into the position it was originally intended for.

Let's get back to the knees for a minute. In our years of training, we have learnt how important it is to keep the knees in proper alignment, with the kneecap (patella) moving directly over the first and second toe. One common misalignment of the knees occurs when the knees collapse in towards one another, often referred to as knock knees, or genu valgum. In this case, one of the first things we do is to strengthen the outer thigh muscles (i.e. the glutes), in order to get the legs and knees back into better alignment. If the postural position of a client is such that they are unable to properly utilize their glute muscles, like someone with a flat-back posture, then it's possible that the knees will take the brunt of the alignment issues. We have worked with many clients for whom we could see a clear link between their lower-back posture and their lower-limb alignment.

In his original work *Return to Life*, Joseph Pilates outlines the 34 mat exercises he wants you to do daily. However, a majority of these exercises are performed in this posterior-pelvis position, with the butt tucked underneath the spine, and the abdominals kept very tight. Once again, we will outline and prescribe exercises we believe will help move the pelvis into a more neutral position, activate the glutes and create a better overall function in the body. We pay homage to Uncle Joe by making slight adjustments to his original work in order to cater to the postural adjustments that modern society now requires. We relish the fact that the Pilates world has embraced this philosophy, and that these adjustments to his work are in line with what Uncle Joe would have wanted.

ASSESSMENT:

- Stand normally and place your hands in a triangle position, with your fingers touching and your thumbs touching.
- Place this triangle on your stomach area, with your fingertips touching your pubic bone, and your thumbs below your belly button.
- Look down at your hand. Are your fingers protruding forward more than your thumbs? If so, then your pubic bone is more forward than your pelvis, which means you have a flat-back posture.

Why Bother?

Those with a flat-back posture also battle the 'wide butt' image. Without the curvature in the lower back (or 'dinner' portion of your spine), the gluteus maximus muscles are not developed, and therefore the butt has the appearance of looking wide rather than rounded. This posture also compresses the waist area, providing little to no 'hourglass' shape. As mentioned earlier, this posture is usually combined with hunchback and therefore, the large C shape of the body shortens the stance. If the potential knee and back pain isn't bad enough, the shorter, wider appearance of your body should be enough to motivate you into alignment.

What if I Have a Perfect Posture?

Some people are born with a more natural alignment and can sustain it better. Others pay attention to it more often and therefore don't have major alignment issues. Either way, if you found that you passed all three assessments with flying colours, then, great job! Of course, we will recommend Pilates for you to help maintain your posture and to help tone and trim your body. The other benefits, such as breath control and muscle toning, are amazing and you will fall in love with how Pilates makes you feel inside out. In Chapter 8, we will suggest exercises depending on your assessments above. If you found no major postural deviations, then when you arrive at Chapter 8, we suggest you do a workout with *all* of the exercises listed. You can do all twenty described in the chapter, or you can pick any number of exercises in any order. Chapter 9 will suggest workouts you can do that include all the exercises; these workouts are perfect for you.

Coming Up Next

We hope you've taken a moment to do the assessments and
determine your postural issues. Most people have a hunchback
posture to a certain degree, but the postural deviations of the
lower body vary from person to person. Now that you've
determined what you would like to work on in terms of your
body shape, the exercises in Chapter 8 will help you address
these issues. However, before we get there, we would like to
dedicate some time to proper nutrition. Without good food
intake, your body will not change the way you want it to.
Proper fuel will result in proper function and get you ready to
add a Pilates workout regime to your daily routine.

SHAPE YOUR EATING HABITS

*The man who uses intelligence with respect to his diet,
his sleeping habits, and who exercises properly, is beyond
any question of a doubt taking the very best preventative
medicines provided so freely and abundantly by nature.*
Joseph Pilates, *Return to Life through Contrology*

In a previous chapter, we mentioned the terms 'breakfast',
'lunch' and 'dinner' as references for the spine. However, the
real breakfast, lunch and dinner are also important in making
sure you look your best.

You wake up in the morning and race to get to the office
or to school. Maybe you grab a muffin from Starbucks on the
way; maybe you skip it. For lunch, you are treated to pizza at
an event and perhaps, for dinner, your family visits the local
Chinese restaurant, and you indulge on a late-night feast of
noodles and rice. Sounds familiar? If so, you are not alone.

All the Pilates exercises in the world will not be able to
combat the caramel popcorn you ate at the movies, the French
fries you ate for lunch or the ice cream for dessert. You can
do the daily exercises, stand taller and create a better-looking
body; however, the fat layer over your stomach area will
not dissipate until you start eating correctly. So let's have

47

a real talk about real food and break it down so it is easy to understand and simple to follow. Be advised, we are not nutritionists; however, we have a combined twenty-five-plus years of experience advising people on what to put into their bodies to complement the perfect workout.

Most people tend to participate in the see-food diet. This is when you eat everything you see! It's easy to do this because food is central to our culture and the focus of many family and religious gatherings. Cooking and feeding people are ways in which we show love and affection for our friends and family. Processed foods are starting to make their way into our culture, as are fast-food chains. Have you ever visited a buffet? These are not designed for you to eat everything in sight. A buffet is meant to cater to a variety of people, and if you plan to eat everything in the buffet, you are going to overeat.

A friend once told me a great story about his relationship with food. When he was younger, he struggled financially to feed himself and couldn't afford to eat the foods he wanted. Now that he is older and can afford to buy himself as much food as he desires, he *still* cannot eat all the food he wants. That's ironic, isn't it? The reality is, your relationship with food can change so that you eat plenty of healthy choices, and on occasion (and in moderation), still treat yourself.

If fat loss is your goal, then what you need is to implement a simple math equation: calories ingested into your body must be less than calories burned by your body. Weight-loss food plans are designed to place the body in a 200–500 calorie deficit so that in a week, your body will shed weight. It takes a deficit of 7700 calories to burn off one kilo of fat. As you can see, burning a kilo of fat will take consistency and perseverance.

If you want to maintain your body weight, then caloric input must equal caloric output. If you work out on a certain day, or climb a mountain and ride a bike, you are able to consume more calories. If you lay in bed sick all day, then your food intake should be less. Maintaining balance, using this simple energy equation throughout your whole life, is the ultimate challenge. Over a lifetime, it is hard to remain consistent as you experience life events such as child bearing, hormone fluctuations, activity changes and constant food cravings. So we will break down all the elements needed to help you understand when to eat, what to eat and how to eat.

Sports Nutritionist Kinita Kadakia Patel on Eating Right

In an ideal world, everyone would work out just enough and eat just right all of the time. In a perfect world, we could just eat what we wanted and not have to work out at all.

Sadly, we all know that's just a fantasy.

So, as a sports nutritionist who lives in the real world, I know we all need to put in at least a little bit of work. And that means the right combination of eating right and exercising right.

I recommend Pilates to most of my clients to achieve their goals because it conditions the entire body; no muscle group is over or undertrained. Your entire musculature is evenly balanced and conditioned, helping you enjoy daily activities and sports with greater ease, better performance and less chance of injury.

When to Eat

When you wake up in the morning, we urge you to start your day with two glasses of warm water. The first purpose of this is to rehydrate your body after eight to nine hours of sleep-fasting. The body is 60 per cent water, and without enough water, the function of your organs will begin to slow down. Your metabolism also slows down because the brain thinks that maybe you can't find water, and as a result, the body moves into survival mode and increases fat storage. That's right! Your body will hold on to the fat since it's not sure what is going on out there in the big, bad world. The second reason for these glasses of water is satiation. Satiety, or the feeling of being full, is important when you are embarking on a plan to lose weight. The fuller you feel all day, the less you will eat.

Why warm? It's easier to drink water warm than cold. We recommend adding some lemon to the water to increase the liver's toxin flush, and add in a drop or two of honey to help offset the taste of the lemon. Whip this up as soon as you awake, and then move right on to breakfast.

Much like the fact that dehydration forces your body into starvation mode, triggering fat retention, skipping breakfast does the exact same thing. The body needs fuel to move, much like a car needs petrol to move. Without fuel, the engine starts to shut down. Breakfast is your most important meal, and must be eaten within thirty minutes of waking up. A solid, balanced breakfast such as oatmeal or an egg-white omlette should be eaten before you work out, sit down at your desk, take the kids to school, or any other activity that begins your day. Eat breakfast. Always.

After your healthy breakfast, you must plan to eat something every 2–3 hours. This helps fuel your body all day long, supporting the calories you burn off with healthy calories coming in. This will prevent you from getting overly hungry and overeating. Eating breakfast will help prevent you from feeling like you are on any 'diet'. Eat frequently, eat often and eat well.

Proper Eating Times

Everyone's life and schedule are different; therefore, it's impossible to tell you exactly when to eat. However, here is a suggested regimen based on a schedule of waking up at 7 a.m. and going to sleep at 11 p.m.:

7.00 a.m.: Wake up
7.30 a.m.: Breakfast (must eat within thirty minutes of waking)
10.00 a.m.: Snack one
12.30 p.m.: Lunch
3.00 p.m.: Snack two
5.30 p.m.: Snack three
8.30 p.m.: Dinner (must not eat less than two hours before sleeping)
11.00 p.m. Sleep

We will outline some sample nutrition plans later in this chapter, which are plans that we specifically use for some of our more famous clients. You will notice we have broken down each plan into 5–6 meals. This is in keeping with our mission to eat often in small quantities and fuel the body throughout the day. We also urge you to stop eating at least two hours before you plan to go to bed. There is no reason to add fuel to your body when you are about to go into hibernation mode and your activity for the day is behind you.

What to Eat

It's not just the calories that make a difference to how you look; it's what kind of calories you consume that makes a difference. Someone who eats a thousand calories a day in doughnuts and ice cream will look and feel entirely different from someone who eats a thousand calories a day in veggies, proteins and wholegrains. The first person will be lacking in nutrients and muscle mass, and will probably look fatter and sloppier. The other person will be leaner, healthier and smaller all around. Which would you like to be?

We must also mention that each food item has a certain calorie quantity associated with it. For example, a gram of protein is equal to four calories, a gram of carbohydrate is four and a gram of fat is nine. Yes, you read that correctly. Fat has more than double the calories than protein and carbohydrates. For this reason, and many others, we encourage you to pay attention to the amount of fat that you consume. We will also emphasize the importance of eating the correct kind of carbohydrate, essentially staying away from items that convert into sugar in the body. Despite the lower caloric value of four calories per gram, sugary carbohydrates can wreak havoc on appetite and overall wellness.

Eat Your Veggies!

First, let's concentrate on vegetables. These should be the lifeblood of our diet. They are nutrient-dense, loaded with fibre to help with digestion, low in calories and amazing for your hair, skin and nails. Eat your vegetables first. Eat a salad before you eat the rest of your meal. Fill your stomach up with the nutrients and fibre that vegetables will offer you before you move on to other items on your plate. Eat a vegetable at every meal. 'Even for breakfast?' you ask. Why not? I (Zeena) will sometimes eat salad for breakfast. This may not be your choice but a veggie egg-white omelette, or a veggie-loaded sambar can help satisfy this requirement.

Let's talk about two 'vegetables' that shouldn't be in every meal: corn and potatoes. While corn is technically a fruit, the way that it is processed and digested in your body can make it seem more like a carbohydrate. The same goes for potatoes. While they are both healthy foods that come from the earth, when attempting to lose weight and get leaner, they should be eaten in moderation.

The best vegetables to consume on a regular basis are the green, leafy kind. These provide a powerhouse of fibre and nutrients, and do a wonderful job filling you up.

Protein for Muscles

The next important item on your plate at every meal should be protein. For vegetarians and meat eaters alike, protein is important in keeping you satiated. The main reason we should be concerned with protein intake is its role in rebuilding muscles after a workout. The reality behind muscle-strengthening workouts is that we are actually 'tearing' the muscle fibres so that they can regenerate and build back stronger. Protein in your diet will aid in the rebuilding and maintenance of your muscles.

My Protein May Be Incomplete

There is a difference between the kinds of protein you ingest. Animal-based proteins are usually called 'complete proteins', which means that it has all the essential amino acids. Some plant-based proteins are 'incomplete proteins', which usually means that they are missing an amino acid. Combining two or more incomplete proteins can make a complete protein, so for vegetarians, this is very important to know and understand.

Here is a list of plant-based foods that contain complete protein. Please note that many of these foods will not be categorized as 'protein' in this book. Some are veggies and some are 'fats', but we are listing these for vegetarians who are interested in foods that will provide them with all the essential amino acids:

Amaranth
Pumpkin seeds
Quinoa
Buckwheat
Hemp seeds
Chia seeds
Spirulina

Here is a list of plant-based incomplete proteins:

Nuts
Seeds
Legumes
Grains
Vegetables

Have you ever heard the phrase 'muscle weighs more than fat'? Well, it's a rather silly phrase, because a kilo of muscle will weigh exactly the same as a kilo of fat. But the difference is that a kilo of muscle is much smaller and denser than the equal amount of fat. So if you are comparing a seventy-kilo person who has 25 per cent fat in their body, with a seventy-kilo person who has 15 per cent fat in their body, it is clear that the second person will look smaller and fitter.

In addition to this, muscle actually burns six times more calories than fat. If you are looking to increase your metabolism, you are essentially looking to increase the amount of calories your body burns on a daily basis. The seventy-kilo person with only 15 per cent body fat will naturally have more muscle mass and, therefore, faster metabolism. This means that when the leaner person eats ice cream or a samosa, their body will burn it much faster than the person with 75 per cent body fat (and less muscle).

There is no greater argument for making sure you have enough protein in your diet than a discussion on the role of protein in aiding and assisting you in building enough muscle in your body.

Women often say, 'I don't want to look big and bulky like a man.' Well, rest assured, it is incredibly difficult to build muscles in a woman's body equivalent to those in a man's. Men have testosterone, which naturally supports muscle growth. Have you ever wondered why it's often easier and faster for your husband, brother or father to lose weight? Their added muscle mass contributes to that higher metabolism, and faster fat burning. So, unless you plan to pop testosterone pills, the extra muscle that women gain will only add to a nice, lean and toned body. This is especially true if you are doing Pilates.

What proteins should you eat? This depends entirely on your diet. Are you a vegetarian? If so, then your focus will be on tofu, legumes and a variety of beans. If you eat meat, then chicken, turkey and fish should be high on your list. For meat eaters, we recommend a moderate intake of red meat due to its high-caloric nature and excess of saturated fat (the bad kind of fat). Cheese and yogurt are also technically considered proteins, and small quantities of these items are acceptable— but only small portions, since certain kinds of cheese can also be very high in calories and fat.

Make Your Grains Whole

So far, you know that you need veggies and protein on your plate for each of your three main meals. What else can you add to make you feel full and happy? Wholegrains. Note that we said 'wholegrains'. Grains can be confusing, especially as more processed grains like bread, bagels, crackers and tortilla chips flood the market. In this case, we prefer non-processed wholegrains such as brown rice, millet and quinoa. Unprocessed wholegrains digest slowly in the system and help you feel full. Wholegrains are also loaded with fibre, which aids the digestive process. Processed grains have less fibre and are more quickly converted to sugar by your body. Foods that do not contain wholegrains, but have enriched flour in them and appear to be processed, can spike your blood sugar. What goes up must come down, and when the blood sugar crashes, you will crave more sugary items. Even though processed carbohydrates don't taste like sugar, they act like it in the body, so you will go eat more tortilla chips, and the endless cycle continues. Also, sugar can act as an opiate-like substance in the brain which means that it has addictive qualities. Have you ever wondered why it's hard to put down the Doritos after just one chip? Your mind is not tricking you; your food is. So stick with wholegrains and non-processed foods; your waistline, your gut and your liver will thank you.

Here are some examples of wholegrain foods. Eat them!

Quinoa
Brown rice
Millet
Barley
Buckwheat
Bulgur
Farro
Kamut
Oats
Rye
Spelt
Wild rice

Here are some examples of processed foods. Don't eat these!

Tortilla chips
Bread

Cookies
Cake
Potato chips
Biscuits
Papad
White Rice
Store-bought naan/roti

The Skinny on Fat

Now that we are eating a healthy protein- carbohydrate-and wholegrain-filled meal, let's cut the fat out of fat. It is important we talk about the 'good' fats and the 'bad' fats, and just as important to keep it simple. When we look closer at foods primarily made of fat, the ones that come from a plant (avocado, nuts and vegetable oils) are called 'unsaturated fats' and are much better for you than those that come from an animal (primarily, red meat, cheese and milk) called 'saturated fats'.

Saturated fat is also called a 'solid fat', which means it's solid at room temperature. These are animal products such as meat, fish, eggs and dairy. Also, tropical oils such as coconut oil and palm oil have saturated fat.

Unsaturated fat is usually a liquid (oil) and is much better for you. The unsaturated-fat category is broken down into polyunsaturated fat, and is found in most vegetable oils. Ever heard of omega-3 and omega-6 fatty acids? These are also your polyunsaturated fats and are found in seafood and fish. Monounsaturated fats (which are also in the category of unsaturated fats) are found in avocados, nuts, olives and peanut oils.

Trans fats are not naturally occurring but artificially produced, and can be found on labels as 'partially hydrogenated oils'. These fats are present in processed food and are not good for you at all, as they have been proven to increase your chances of coronary heart disease. Much like avoiding processed food for the lack of wholegrains, and high-sugar value, processed foods should also be avoided for the trans fats.

We mentioned oil just now, and it's important to note the role of oil in our diets. Olive oil is a good unsaturated fat, which is important for the cells in our bodies to work effectively. We use olive oil to cook and fry many popular foods in the Indian diet. We also use ghee and coconut oil, which are technically saturated fats, but have been reported to have many health benefits. Unfortunately, despite the fact that oils and ghee are made up of good fats, the overuse of oil and ghee can contribute to an excess of calories. Remember, each gram of fat consists of nine calories, as opposed to the four calories in protein and carbohydrates. You now know that it is important to eat fewer calories than you burn. So keep in mind that a small teaspoon of olive oil contains the same amount of calories as an entire plateful of broccoli. Oil and fats are calorie-dense. Instead of using too much oil, we recommend learning how to cook certain items with veggie/ chicken stock. Try it! Stir-fry some veggies over the stove in chicken stock and spices, and you will end up with a very tasty dish without all the calories. Poaching is a great way to cook without the fat from cooking oils; however, it's important that you enjoy what you are eating, so the cooking method is often a personal preference. If you are trying to lose weight, we recommend staying away from all oils, ghee or coconut oil.

In order to get these good fats, we recommend better options such as avocados and nuts. Avocados are a wonderful addition to the healthy salad you make at lunch, and they make your salad more filling. A variety of nuts, in small, healthy portions, can make a great snack in between meals. Ensure, however, that these nuts are raw as opposed to toasted or roasted. Roasted nuts can be high in salt and sodium, which can create bloating and cause you to retain water.

Get Fruity!

Last, but certainly not least, is fruit. We love fruit for its fibre, sweet taste and amazing nutrients. We encourage fruit as a substitute for anything else sweet you might be craving during the day. Fruits are wonderful with nuts as a snack, and great to add into a smoothie for a midday treat. The fibre in the fruit counteracts the negative effects of sugar on the body.

We don't want to tell anyone not to eat fruit; there are many diet plans out there that condemn certain fruits for their higher sugar content. We love the nutrients found in fruits and believe that if the rest of your diet is balanced, you can choose whatever fruits you want. However, if there is an overload of sugar in your overall diet, then we recommend you avoid the higher-sugar fruits such as bananas, and instead choose lower-sugar fruits such as raspberries and blueberries.

High-Sugar and Low-Sugar Fruits

We adore fruit. The nutrients and fibre in them are excellent additions to your diet. But if you are trying to lose weight, watching your sugar intake can be key.

Here is a list of higher-sugar fruits to avoid:

Tangerines
Cherries
Grapes
Pomegranates
Mangos
Figs
Bananas

Here is a list of lower-sugar fruits that we hope you incorporate into your diet:

Berries
Nectarines
Papaya
Watermelon
Apples

A Plan for You

Here it is: a simple plan, with columns of food laid out for you. Certain foods, such as nuts, often span two categories (protein and fat). Use the list below to help you plan what food would fall into what category for the sake of proper meal planning. You can place the meals and snacks in any order you wish.

Meal one (breakfast): Veggies, Protein, Wholegrain, Fat (minimal)

Snack one: (pick one) Fruit, Veggies, Protein, Fat (minimal)

Meal two (lunch): Veggies, Protein, Wholegrain, Fat (minimal)

Snack two: (pick one) Fruit, Veggies, Protein, Fat (minimal)

Meal three (dinner): Veggies, Protein, Wholegrain, Fat (minimal)

Snack three: (pick one) Fruit, Veggies, Protein, Fat (minimal)

A Quick Recap

Veggies:

Kale

Collard Greens

Swiss Chard

Spinach

Broccoli

Romaine Lettuce

Cabbage

Brussels Sprouts

Alfalfa Sprouts

Peas

Red/Green and Yellow Bell Pepper

Carrot

Squash (technically a fruit)

Tomato (technically a fruit)

Cucumber

Radish
Endive
Eggplant

Protein:

Beans
Legumes
Seeds
Soy
Tofu
Chicken
Turkey
Fish
Beef
Cheese
Natural yogurt (low-sugar)
Cottage cheese
Skimmed milk paneer

Wholegrains:

Quinoa
Brown rice
Millet
Barley
Buckwheat
Bulgar
Farro
Kamut

Oats
Rye
Spelt
Wild rice
Sweet potato (technically a vegetable)

Fat:

Olive/veggie/avocado oil
Nuts
Avocados
Nut butter
Ghee

Fruit:

Apple
Banana
Berries
Pear
Nectarine
Orange
Watermelon
Melon
Papaya
Mango
Grapefruit
Kiwi
Figs
Apricot
Coconut

Pineapple
Lemon
Lime

How Much to Eat

This is the ultimate question. How many calories should I eat in a day? There is a simple calculation you can do to determine a basic resting metabolic rate (The number of calories you burn at rest). The problem is that there are so many variables to this calculation, such as how much muscle you have, that it is often inaccurate. Instead of having you count calories down to the last one, we would rather improve on the foods you are eating, increase the frequency at which you eat, and teach you how to listen to your body. There are some basic guidelines, however, on the portion size that we can suggest to you. This method works well because you can use the palm of your hand to measure how much you eat; clearly, a bigger person will have a bigger palm and therefore can usually accommodate a bigger portion. These guidelines are for one portion for one of your meals listed above.

- Veggies: eat as many as you want and often as you want, as long as they are not coated or cooked/fried in fat.
- Protein: Keep meat and bean portions within the size of the palm of your hand per serving. Keep cheese portions within the size of your thumb per serving.
- Wholegrain: Keep grain portions within the size of your fist per serving.
- Fat: Keep oil to less than a tablespoon a day. Keep nuts to half of the palm of your hand a day. Do not consume more than half an avocado a day.
- Fruit: Consume cut-fruit portions the size of your fist, or one small full piece of fruit per serving.

A Few Important Notes

There are a few other details to be aware of when on a mission to lose weight:

Scrutinize Your Salad Dressing

You can consume all the salads you want, but if you load them with dressings that are terribly high in calories, you will get nowhere. We advise you to choose a lower-calorie dressing that doesn't have too much oil, sugar or dairy. Home-made vinaigrettes are amazing, especially when combined with herbs such as basil and thyme. Also, when eating out, always order your dressing on the side so that you can control your portions. Another tip: use hummus combined with a little lemon. This is a wonderful way to add protein and fibre to your salad, and fill you up.

Read Your Labels

Be very mindful of labels. Something that says 'wholegrain' may have a few enriched ingredients. If something is 'enriched', it is not at all whole. When choosing grains in your diet, stick with things you can cook at home, like brown rice and quinoa, versus things that are processed, like bread and bagels.

Skip the Sugar

Let's talk about sugar. It's everywhere. It's in your ketchup; it's in your tortilla chips. It's addictive, and the more you eat, the more you crave it. It alters your metabolism, it's terrible for your skin and hair, and it makes you fat. Plain and simple. Put down the cake and pick up the apple.

Corn syrup, or high-fructose corn syrup, is processed sugar that is found in processed food. Some experts believe that increased consumption of high-fructose corn syrup is to blame for the increased waistlines worldwide. Not only does it convert to sugar in your body, it's processed so your body cannot digest it as well as it can natural sugar. The problem is that corn syrup is often hidden in food. It is in condiments such as ketchup, salad dressings, pre-made sauces, crackers, cereals, sodas and many other foods—surprised? And remember, sugar can be addictive.

Artificial sweeteners are not a great choice either; the word 'artificial' is the key indicator here. Despite the 'no sugar, no calories' appeal, there are numerous reports from people around the world linking the use of aspartame with a variety of health problems such as headaches, memory loss and digestive distress. More important, however, is the effect this has on the brain. When we keep tricking our body into thinking that we are eating something sweet, it keeps craving sweet. So you haven't really addressed the root cause of your weight gain: your sweet tooth. Part of the benefit of cutting back on sweet and sugary foods is the change in your palate. Suddenly, fruit becomes sweeter and you can use fruit as a dessert instead of grabbing an artificially-sweetened substitute.

If you *must* eat something sweet, here are our recommendations: the more natural the better. Sweeteners such as agave nectar, honey and jaggery are more natural and can be processed more easily in your system. The only sugar-free sweetener we would recommend is Stevia, which is derived from a plant and is therefore more natural than its chemically-laden counterpart.

How Can I Cut Out the Sugar?

It's scary for most people. We think—if I cut out all the sugars in my body, including some grains and processed foods, won't I go hungry? Won't I be miserable? The tough-love answer is: maybe. It will be hard in the beginning. Your body and your brain are used to these tastes and textures. But after three days, your cravings will minimize and your sweet tooth will begin to subside. After a week, you will notice that you are craving less and less, and you will notice a difference in your waistline. Finally, after three weeks you will eat a piece of fruit and notice that it suddenly tastes different! Wait, how did that apple get so sweet? Is it coated in sugar? No! Your mind and your body have adjusted.

If you're stuck on a plateau and struggling to lose some weight, we recommend cutting down on the wholegrain portion of the diet plan outlined above. Sure, it's whole. Sure, it's better for you than a doughnut. But it still converts to sugar in your body and if you want to achieve your goal, it could be preventing you from making the final drop. Instead, load up on extra vegetables and protein. This is a sure-fire solution to getting leaner in a very safe and healthy way.

Don't Drink Your Calories

You may have the perfect diet, but add three glasses of wine and a margarita and you've just added over 500 calories to your dietary intake. Not to mention, the possible hangover the next day may have you eating French fries to help you recover.

Drinking alcohol can be a deadly obstacle to any weight-loss goal. It adds sugar and calories, and the resulting loss in judgement while drinking can also cause you to overeat. For many people who enjoy a couple of drinks, it is unrealistic to believe that they will stop consuming alcohol for the rest of their life. Therefore, here are some simple guidelines for you to follow when consuming alcohol:

- Choose drinks as low in sugar as possible. The best options are red wine (the label must say less than 11.5 per cent alcohol), light beer and clear, hard alcohol mixed with club soda, water, or on the rocks.

Pass the Screwdrivers

I (Zeena) once had a client early in my career who was aiming to lose over twenty kilos. She wrote in her nutrition diary every day. She would come to the gym more than three times a week, and was very cautious of everything she put in her mouth. She huffed and puffed and whined and complained every week when she would see her weight loss was minimal, or nothing. During one session, she mentioned that her adventures the night before had left her feeling terrible. I asked what she had had to drink and looked in her nutrition journal to see if she had written it down. I was shocked when she admitted to drinking two to four screwdrivers (vodka with orange juice) a night! 'I didn't write it down because it's not food, right?' She was consuming 360–720 calories more than her allotted amount per day! No wonder she wasn't losing weight! We got the drinking under control and taught her how to make smarter choices, and she soon began to shed weight.

- Avoid high-sugar mixers at all costs.
- Drink a glass of water in between each glass in order to minimize dehydration and 'hangover' effects the next day, and avoid overeating.
- Take time between each drink to assess where you are and make sure not to overeat during the evening.
- Make sure you eat a light meal consisting of protein before you start drinking. This is to avoid hunger pangs and munching on unhealthy starters at parties.

How to Eat

Now that you know the essentials of how best to eat to maximize fat loss, it's important to consider the thought process behind how to eat. Eating well consistently, seven days a week, 365 days a year, can be difficult at first. We are not going to lie to you about this—it is hard. You will need to use one of your new Pilates principles: concentration. Your mind will need to focus on what you put in your mouth, and when to put it in your mouth. However, over time, it does get easier, and you will begin to see great results. Before you know it, your new eating habits will become second nature. At first, it's difficult to remember not to chow down on the samosa lying in your mother's kitchen, or indulge in ice cream with your children. Over time, it will become a habit to order a salad at the pizza place. It will become second nature to skip the fried appetizers and focus on the main dish of protein and fibre. You will suddenly crave two glasses of water when you wake up. And you will become so accustomed to eating every 2–3 hours that your body will get hungry even if you don't. Over time, it will become natural and easy. But in the beginning, you will have to concentrate.

We highly recommend that you always sit down while eating. Driving while eating, talking on the phone and pacing while eating, or eating while walking to the gym, all distract you from paying attention to what you eat. Paying attention to what you eat is the same as concentrating on what you eat and how fast you eat it. We recommend you chew slowly while you eat. Taking your time while chewing allows your central nervous system to process your food and eventually tell your mind when you are full.

Mindful Eating

When mealtime comes, you pick up the spoon, place it in your mouth and chew. Right? Sounds simple, but often, we aren't concentrating on what we eat at the moment we are eating it. We would like to introduce you to something called 'mindful eating'. This helps you create more awareness about what you place in your mouth. Here is an example of what could happen when you are engaged in eating mindfully:

You pick up a spoonful of food. You take a look at it. What does it smell like? What do you think it will feel like in your mouth? Will you chew it carefully or instantly swallow it? These are all amazing questions to ask yourself just before you put your fuel into your body. Wow! That was an explosion of flavours, you think to yourself. Or maybe the bite was too hot or too cold. Or perhaps you decide your next bite needs an extra sprinkle of salt. Your mind is talking out loud and you are pausing to process what it thinks before you move on to the next bite. Finally, you are starting to look at an emptier plate. Your companions have wolfed down their food and are waiting for you. You think to yourself, maybe I'm full, there's no need to finish, I will take my leftovers home. You pause for 5 minutes, confirm your diagnosis, and move on. Minutes later, dessert gets placed on the table. It is your favourite dessert. You are full, but your mind is reminding you how yummy it tastes and how amazing it will feel on your tongue. You

Indulgence versus Satisfaction

I (Yasmin) had a client who came to me needing to lose twenty kilos as soon as possible. She was going to be featured in a movie soon, and it was of utmost importance that she look her best. The problem was, she was so hungry all the time! I had her write down her food intake for me because I believe that each person's food plan should be unique. It became quite clear that she had been overindulging for years. She would eat until she was beyond full; therefore, her stomach was used to being fed large quantities. I gave her a food plan that was six smaller meals a day, advising her to eat until just *before* she felt full. I told her that ten minutes after she was done eating, her stomach would feel the effects of her eating and become full. Of course, this was very difficult for her at first, and she was quite uncomfortable. However, she ended up losing 2.5 kilos in less than twenty days! The results motivated her, and she began to understand that indulgence and satisfaction are two different things. Her stomach and her brain needed to be rewired; they both had to learn what the correct amount of food was in order to properly nourish her body.

pause. You know you shouldn't eat it. You think to yourself: 'Is a bite of this special treat going to be worth the after-effect of overeating, the physiological sugar responses and the mental guilt?' You decide that what you want now (the dessert) is not more important than what you want forever (health). You take a bite to savour the flavour. You put the fork down. And you repeat to yourself: 'What I want to look and feel like is more important than what I want to put in my mouth right now.'

This is mindful eating. Be mindful of everything you put into your body.

It's important to remember that there are many temptations to shut down your mind and simply stuff food into your mouth. Food is everywhere. Temptation is everywhere. Stop. Be mindful. Remind yourself of what you want most. Remind yourself of what you want forever.

Coming Up Next

All calories are not created equal: there are good ones and bad ones. Eat protein to build muscle and increase your metabolism. Eat vegetables to load up on fibre and essential nutrients for brain and body function. Fuel your body every few hours. Eat mindfully. These are a few easy tips to assist you with your new Pilates routine and help you look leaner in you new posture. In the next chapter, we will introduce you to poor movement patterns in the way that many people sit, stand, sleep and walk. We will discuss how these poor movement patterns can affect your posture. Embarking on getting fit involves changing many things in your life, including the way you move through it every day.

SHAPE YOUR EVERYDAY LIFE

With body, mind and spirit functioning perfectly as a coordinated whole, what else could reasonably be expected other than an alert, disciplined person?
Joseph Pilates, *Return to Life through Contrology*

Unlike our inspiration Uncle Joe, we will not tell you how to bathe. We assume you're quite an expert at that one! However, we do have some other wisdom to impart in the area of general living that can influence how successful you are in building a life of health and happiness. We see our clients for 2—maybe 3—hours a week. The other 165 hours when they are not with us, some of them mess up everything we have worked to achieve. To help with this, we give homework similar to the strategies we outline below, and we ask clients to pay attention to what they do outside their Pilates practice.

Sitting, standing, walking and sleeping take up a significant portion of our day. Creating new awareness about the way you go through these movements can have a powerful impact. We have had clients who walk in complaining of either lower back or knee pain. When we evaluate their posture, we find that they have unbalanced hips, and they eventually admit to sitting cross-legged at their desk, or lying too much on the same side when they sleep or watch TV. Sometimes, we will notice someone who always stands with their weight loaded on one leg, with a hip jutting out. Or perhaps when they walk they are always leaning and favouring one side. Asking them to make simple changes can alter the way their body moves and therefore reduce their pain significantly.

Ileana D'Cruz and Her Love for Pilates

Okay, first things first: I hate going to the gym! The thought of lifting weights and running on a treadmill is not at all appealing to me. I've always wanted to get fit but all the traditional training techniques just bored me. Also, I've got a tricky body type to deal with and it's always been hard for me to tone up those problem areas (yes, ladies, you know I'm talking about a jiggly butt and thighs) and strengthen my body; also, I wanted to do all this without getting bulky.

So when Yasmin introduced me to Pilates, I was intrigued and curious. It looked interesting—very different from the other kinds of workouts I had tried before. Let me just say, I love going to the gym now! Pilates has helped strengthen my core immensely; it also helped better my posture. I felt healthier and more energized, and my body has never looked better than it does now. I saw results in just a month! All I do now is Pilates. I love that there are different machines you can use and different kinds of exercises. I can do a new workout every day! I think it is the perfect fit for me. Yasmin introduced a whole new way for me to get fit and I love it! You don't need to lift heavy weights and run for hours to get a great, strong, toned body; Pilates does it all and so much better. There are days when my body just feels sore and tired and doing a session of Pilates stretches it out and makes me feel great and rejuvenated.

Hunters and Gatherers

In Chapter 1, we referenced a study done in 2013 amongst Indian IT professionals, in which over 50 per cent of them reported incidences of lower back pain. How is it possible that more than half of this population is in chronic pain? If you look at our ancestry and how humans survived many years ago, everyone lived off the land, and hunted and gathered their food. We lifted and pushed and pulled and yanked and did everything physical in our daily life. We didn't write or read much but spent the days working towards the next meal and the next night of sleep. As civilization developed, we advanced to this new computer generation and our bodies have not adjusted as well to our new movement patterns. It's a rather new discovery for us since this modern-day culture of sitting at desks for hours on end has only developed over the last 30–40 years. Clearly, sitting with our hips in flexion, our pelvis tucked under and our head leaning forward for hours on end is not what our bodies were originally designed for.

How to Sit

It's sitting down for hours at a time that got us humans into this mess in the first place. We were designed to be hunters and gatherers, not typists and texters. Our bodies were never meant to sit for hours on end in an extreme hip-flexion position. The hip flexors, which are the muscles that run across the front of the thigh bone and into the pelvis, or the hamstrings which run along the back of the thighs, can become chronically tight. This tightness contributes to arched back or flat-back postures as described in Chapter 2.

More importantly, sitting for hours can drain the energy and circulation from our bodies. Muscles become atrophied, and when these muscles lose their size and strength, they begin to impact our posture negatively. We get lazy from the fatigue and this fatigue comes from lack of movement. It can turn into a vicious cycle.

So how should you sit? Firstly, don't sit for prolonged periods of time. Stand up, take a break, walk around your desk, lift you arms and stretch. Also, be sure that the positioning of your chair is correct. Are you able to sit up straight without rounding your lower back into the chair? If not, use a small lower back support to try to get into this position. It is important that your lower back has a small arch in it when you sit. Without this arch, your lower back muscles will become strained, and your hamstrings will become extremely tight. You should be able to feel the two bony parts of your butt under you—the sitz bones. If you can't feel your sitz bones under you, chances are your pelvis is not in the correct position.

Be careful to avoid the common sitting position where one leg is crossed directly over the other. Most women sit this way; perhaps we were taught by our great grandmothers that this is the way to sit 'like a lady'. But common sense tells us that this position can create imbalances in the hips and spine. Just think, when you sit with the right leg crossed directly over the left, with the right butt muscle stretched longer, the right inner thigh is shortened, and the right hip is rotated forward. If you do this over and over again, for hours on end, your body will take this position and create muscle memory around them. The repetition of this common habit, and the resulting muscle memory, could be a cause of pain due to muscular imbalances.

Lastly, and most importantly, you must be able to sit up straight, with a straight upper back, and your eyes must be looking forward. A majority of issues related to kyphosis (or hunchback posture) occur as a result of sitting for hours, staring at your phone or computer, and allowing the shoulders to round forward. We would like to recommend a few exercises that can be done at your desk or computer station, to assist in combating this hunchback posture. Setting a simple alarm on your phone or computer can remind you to do these exercises a few times a day.

Shoulder Rolls

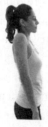 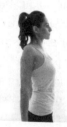

Shoulder roll begins   Shoulder roll ends

Sit tall with your sitz bones firmly planted in your chair. Lift your shoulders up to your ears and then roll them back. Imagine there is a pencil between your two scapula (shoulder blades), and gently squeeze the pencil. Do these shoulders rolls and scapula squeezes at least 5 times, 3 times a day.

Towel Squeeze

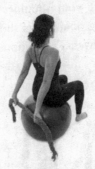

Stand up with a towel or Thera-Band in your hands behind your back, with your hands as close to each other as possible. Keep the arms straight and your palms facing backwards. Keeping your shoulders back, and your elbows straight, pull the towel/band apart for 2 seconds and hold, then release. Repeat this 5 times, 3 times a day.

Shoulder Openers

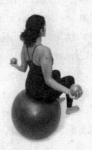

Stand with your upper arms glued to your sides, your elbows bent and your palms face-up. Hold on to something heavy in each hand (equal weight—maybe two water bottles). Keeping your upper arms by your sides, rotate the arms open and apart, while squeezing your shoulder blades together, then return to your starting point. This shoulder-blade squeeze is super-important. Do twenty repetitions, three times a day.

Side Stretch

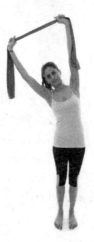

Stand up with a towel or Thera-Band in your hands, the distance between them a little wider than your shoulder width. Bring your arms up straight above your head with the towel/band pulled tight. Lean your body over to the left as you stretch your right side. Keep a tight grip on the towel/band, keep your elbows soft and attempt to keep your shoulders down and away from your ears. Hold this for a minimum of thirty seconds on each side, once a day.

Simple Solution

I (Zeena) had a client who went back to work with her son after a three-year break. She was thrilled to be working in a place with someone she loved and trusted. Except, she had one problem: her neck was in terrible pain—so much so that she stopped working out and was gaining weight! She consulted a doctor who gave her prescription medication for the pain and a chiropractor who treated her—and these things helped—but two days later, the pain came back. Finally, I asked her: 'How are you sitting at your desk?' She replied with a meandering explanation of how she used a tiny laptop and moved around from desk to desk, using whatever was available to her. In that moment, she discovered her own problem: she was becoming more kyphotic from rounding forward in her terrible sitting position. We discussed proper sitting habits, found a solution to raise her laptop, and I sent her home with instructions on some simple stretches and exercises—the very ones listed above. Two weeks later, the pain had subsided considerably, and she was able to resume her workouts again.

How to Stand

Similar to walking, standing has become less popular over the years, as driving and sitting have taken over. Those who do stand often do so in high heels or footwear that is highly inappropriate for alignment, making the problems in the body even worse. Our bodies were meant to stand; it's what makes us different from the animals we evolved from. We are meant to be upright, and the organs and tissues in our body all function better when we are upright.

In Chapter 2, we outlined the plumb line: the line that should be drawn from the side of your body through the ear, the shoulder, the hip bone, the knee joint and the ankle. This is the ideal stance for the body in its vertical position. Often, people tend to lean into one hip more than the other. Doing this will create compensatory patterns in your hips. Don't do it! You should stand with weight evenly distributed between both feet as often as you can. What should you do with your arms and hands? Do not cross them in front of you. This perpetuates the hunched shoulders we are trying to avoid (it also gives people the impression that you are trying to hide from them—see Chapter 6 for more information on this concept). Instead, hold your arms down at your side, or grasp your hands behind yourself. The latter position is optimal, since it promotes an opening of the chest and shoulder muscles.

Much like walking and sitting, it's important to create awareness about the way you stand. The following is a simple practice exercise that can be done any time, anywhere, against a stretch of bare wall. Stand with your back against the wall, with your heels directly against the wall. Make sure that your behind is against the wall, but your lower back is not pressed into it. The 'lunch' part of your spine (mid-back/thoracic spine) is up against the wall, as are your shoulders and head. Be sure to keep your eyes looking directly forward at all times. Turn your palms to face forward, with the back of your hands pushing up against the wall. Feel the back of your arms pressing against the wall. If this position is difficult to hold, then walk 2–3 inches forward and assume the same position.

Practise this posture for 2–3 minutes a day. Close your eyes and visualize the impression you are leaving on the wall behind you. Feel the muscles in your back engage and fire up. These are the muscles that will get you re-energized and realigned.

How to Sleep

This section is referring specifically to how you lie down when sleeping at night. Of the 24 hours in your day, ideally, almost 8 of those hours are spent in a lying-down position, either sleeping or resting. How you sleep and what you sleep on is critical to how you feel when you wake up in the morning.

The worst thing to do when lying down is to lie on your stomach. Think about it: when you are lying on your front, it means that your head has to turn to one side or the other to accommodate your face. This means that your cervical spine is constantly rotated and placing pressure on one side of your spine more than the other, for hours on end.

Lying on your side is a better option, though not optimal for the same reasons as above. If you must lie on your side, it's important to have a pillow large enough to support the space between the ear and the shoulder. This is to ensure that the head is in proper alignment and not tilted in either direction, either too high or too low. When lying on your side, you want to make sure the head is centred directly between the shoulders, and the pillow under the bottom ear should be high enough to assist this.

However, as noted, lying on your side for hours on end is not optimal unless you can guarantee that you will switch sides halfway through the night.

Finding the Perfect Pillow

Not long ago, while travelling, I (Yasmin) ventured into the shopping area of the airport, as I often do, only to find a place selling pillows. I am always on the lookout for the perfect pillow, and was amazed to find one that I absolutely loved. It was of an ideal height and provided good support, so despite the high price, I was happy to buy it. My travelling mates laughed at my obsession and joked at the price of something so seemingly unimportant. I explained to them the benefits of using the right pillow, and the implications on their necks and spines from sleeping incorrectly. Six of my friends went on to purchase the same pillow. I almost asked for commissions from the shop owner! A few days later, we all met at a party and everyone seemed happy with their new sleeping companions.

This is because the bottom shoulder gets pushed forward when it's laid upon. Once again, this can create imbalances in the shoulders and ribcage. How can you guarantee that you will switch sides halfway through the night? If you get up to go to the restroom in the middle of the night, this is a great opportunity to change sides. However, it's difficult to make sure this always happens, which is why we recommend the final position: lying on your back.

Lying on your back, as uncomfortable as it might seem, is really the optimal way to sleep. When lying on your back, it mimics the way you stand: your spine is in proper alignment and not contorted in either direction. New ergonomic pillows in the market support this position by placing a bigger lump at the part of the pillow under your neck, and allowing the head to fall back into a more neutral position. If the head is lifted very high on an overabundance of pillows, this actually creates the same 'forward head' position as if you were sitting at a desk. Why would you want to mimic the same position sleeping, that causes you pain while you are sitting? You don't have to! Therefore, the use of these new pillows can help ensure that your neck and spine are aligned for the whole eight hours you are asleep.

Lastly, and most importantly, sleeping on your back can improve your skin. Hours of lying on the side of the face can create wrinkle lines. Sleeping on your back eliminates this and allows your skin and pores to breathe.

Sleep Solutions

I (Zeena) got into Pilates because of my constantly ailing back. I was born with a right leg slightly shorter than the left, which sometimes created pain and imbalances throughout my spine. My Pilates regimen is a required element in keeping me healthy and strong. Years ago, I visited a colleague to help me determine why my ribcage consistently rotated to the left. Even in X-rays, my belly button ring was clearly shown rotated to the left of my spine! In our conversation, he asked how I slept. Aha! I realized that I always slept on my right side, which technically pushed my right shoulder forward and also pushed my whole ribcage to the left. It was a simple explanation for what I thought was a complicated problem, and over time, I have learnt to enjoy sleeping on my back. When I lie down at night, I imagine that stars are above me and that I am staring up at them; I close my eyes and snooze away.

How to Walk

As a baby, we learn how to put one foot in front of the other, but as we get older, the purity of this walking process diminishes. Injuries, repetitive sports patterns, age and posture can all affect how someone walks. So, what happens when we walk? It's a complicated movement of lower-body patterns. First, the right hip flexes to lift the leg, and the right knee bends to bring the leg forward. Then, weight is placed on the striding leg as the body moves onto it, and the force moves through all the leg muscles. Finally, the leg moves backwards into something called 'hip extension', while the other leg begins the same hip flexion—or knee flexion—body weight transfer and hip extension. So on and so forth.

Walking is something we do every day. Watching a client walk is one of the fundamental ways we assess them when they enter the studio. A baby stands up straight, engages its core and walks upright to find its balance. Many adults we see walk with their feet turned out, tail bone tucked under, shoulders hunched, eyes down and torso flexed forward. Their balance is off, and at any moment, they could easily topple over. In essence, these incorrect walking patterns will eventually cause strain on the joints and muscles. Before you know it, the client is saying, 'My back hurts all the time.' Well, we can help you achieve proper form in the studio, but if you continue to walk hunched over and with a shortened stride, your back will never get better.

Over time, the part of the walking process we lose the most is the latter part of the walking motion: the hip extension. This means that the upper part of the thigh should move behind your pelvis as it moves through the gait cycle. There are a few explanations as to why we lose this movement pattern. Firstly, many of us have underutilized our butt and hamstring (behind the thigh) muscles by sitting all day long. These muscles are critical to the hip-extension portion of the walking-gait cycle. If you sit for a living, or drive a lot, this is probably a concern for you.

Secondly, as we age, every muscle in our body gets tighter. We've mentioned the importance of being vertically aligned when you stand up, and this is even more important when you are walking or running. If the muscle in the front of the thigh (the hip flexor) is tight, it makes it nearly impossible for the leg to move into hip extension. Without this critical movement, other muscles such as the calf muscles get tight from underutilization. This creates a vicious cycle: the muscles get tight and the movement becomes more limited, causing the muscles to get even tighter.

How should we walk? We need to use the backs of our legs more. We need to engage our hamstrings and glutes, which span the butt region down to just above the knee on the backside of the body. We need to stand up taller, we need to squeeze our shoulder blades together, and we need to look forward (not down). When moving your legs through the gait cycle, really think about pushing your leg behind you when you walk. Squeeze the butt a little and feel the back of the leg muscle engage. Exaggerate this movement a bit and you will possibly feel new muscles engage while moving through this motion.

Now, let's talk about feet. The feet are at the root of it all, because they are at the bottom of the body. They are meant to work through a full range of motion when you walk. Your toes should bend above the ball of the foot, and the heel should lift up as your leg moves backwards into hip extension. If your feet are tight and inflexible, this movement becomes limited. Since the feet are the base of the body, this dysfunction will carry itself all the way up to the rest of your body.

Many of the exercises prescribed later in this book are aimed at helping you walk better. You will work on gaining more hip extension, stretching the hip flexors and strengthening the back of the legs. However, the more you walk and the more you concentrate on your movement while walking, the better you will become at walking properly.

How to Live

We can tell you what to eat, how to exercise, how to walk and how to sit. But how to live is an entirely different endeavour. Your life is your own and you have complete control over how you choose to live it. You clearly made a choice when you bought this book. You wanted a life of health and happiness. Maybe it was a celebrity who inspired you to look your best, or perhaps your back pain keeps getting worse and you want to do something about it. Regardless of the reason, you made a choice to read this book, and something inspired you to follow a new, healthy regimen. We commend you for this!

As life gets fast-paced and more technology-oriented, and as ambition and competition permeate deeper into our culture, it's important to take a step back and remember what's important in life. We would like to revisit the six principles of Pilates here and, this time, apply them to life in general:

Concentration: Wake up in the morning and concentrate on what it will take to have a good day. A healthy breakfast? A motivating yoga class? Lunch with your best girlfriend? Shopping with your daughter? We have a million thoughts a day. Take a few of these and concentrate on making them happen.

Control: You can't control everything that happens to you. Family gets sick, businesses get busy and friends need help. But you can control how you react to it. Will you let it get you down, or will you control your choices and decide to let the stress go?

Centre: Find the centre of your life. Your family? Your friends? God? Whatever your centre is, open your heart to it and make it the strongest centre it can be.

Flow: Life can be choppy and stressful. Texts, emails and constant media bombardment can make this jumble of thoughts even worse. If you keep jumping from task to task for no rhyme or reason, your efficiency will decrease. Attempt to build a day that flows cohesively. Accomplish one task before you flow to the next. Plan your day so that your energy can flow peacefully and calmly.

Precision: In life, precision speaks of your purpose. What is your purpose in life? Is it to raise the best children? Build a profitable business? Is it your mission to serve God? Are you looking for charitable opportunities? Whatever your purpose, be precise in your actions to accomplish them. Know your purpose and live it.

Breathing: Without breath, there is no life. Your breath can calm you and energize you. It represents life, light, hope and freedom. Breathe.

Coming Up Next

As we mentioned earlier, Pilates is not just a series of exercises; it is a way of life. When you accept this and begin to live it day in and day out, you will become more committed to living a healthier and happier life. We've discussed proper sitting habits, as well as how to stand tall and walk properly. However, none of this is possible without the power of our own breath. Without the ability to breathe properly, life is stilted and stressed. Proper breath control is one of the primary principles of Pilates and we've dedicated an entire chapter to teaching you how to inhale and exhale, deeply and effectively.

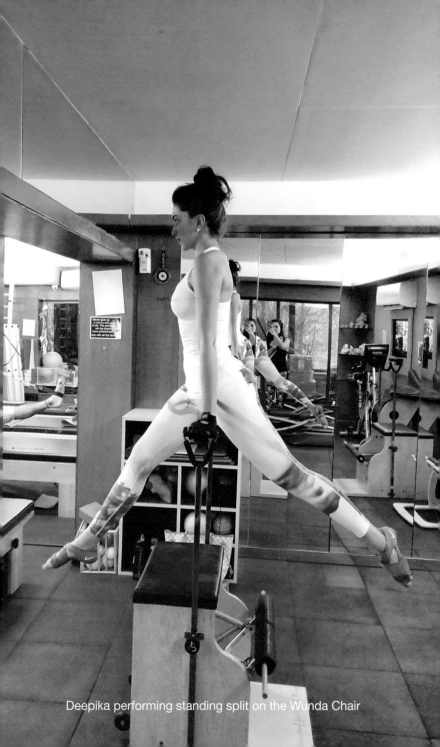

Deepika performing standing split on the Wunda Chair

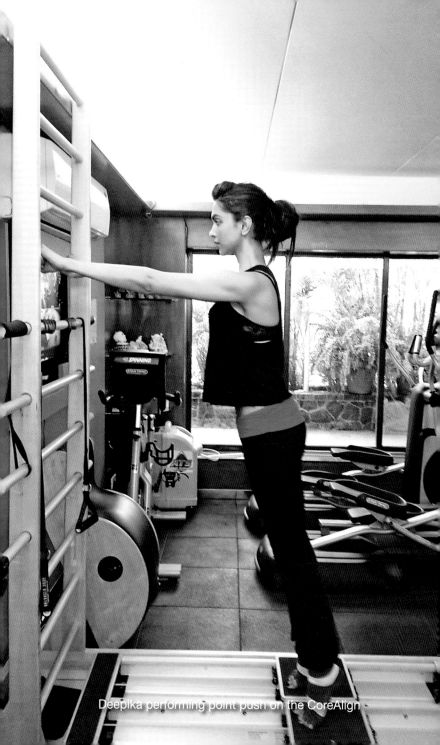

Deepika performing point push on the CoreAlign

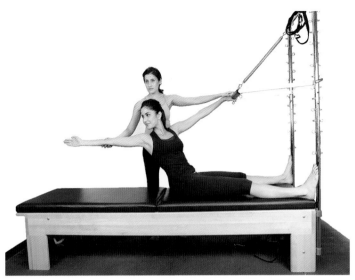

Katrina performing side reach on the Trapeze Table (Cadillac)

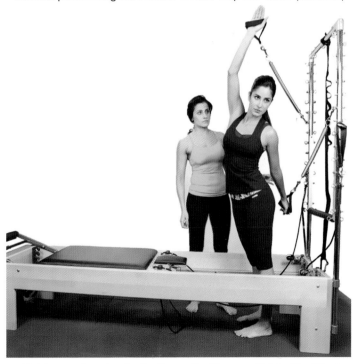

Katrina performing butterfly on the Trapeze Table (Cadillac)

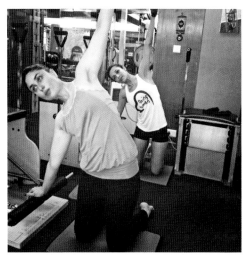

Kareena and Malaika performing side bend
on the Wunda Chair

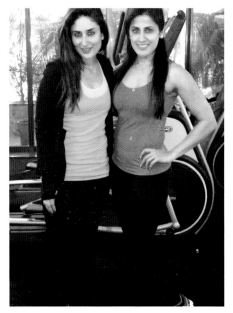

With Kareena—someone who's been there
throughout Yasmin's fitness journey

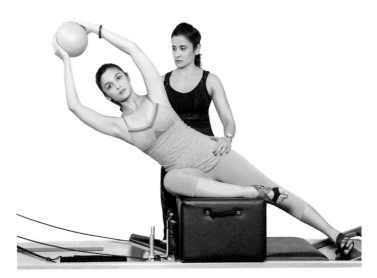

Alia performing side bend over a box on the Reformer

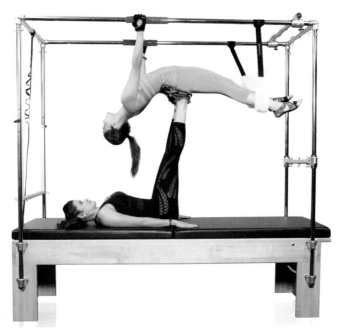

Alia hanging from the Trapeze Table (Cadillac)

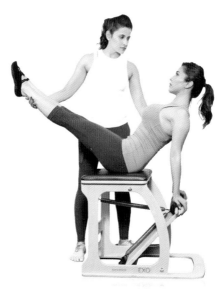

Sophie performing teaser on the Wunda Chair

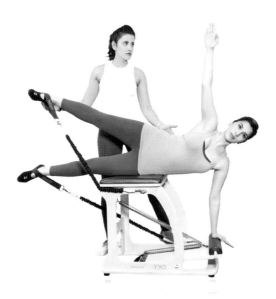

Sophie performing side-lying obliques on the Exo Chair

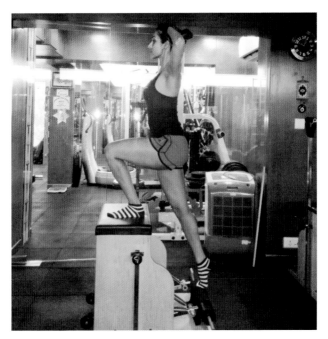

Malaika performing forward lunge on the Wunda Chair

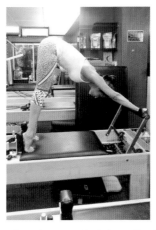

Malaika performing up-stretch on the Reformer

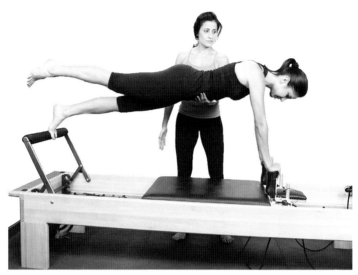

Katrina performing control front, one leg off

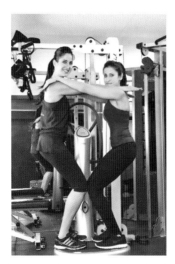

It's always good to have some
fun after a hard Pilates session!

SHAPE YOUR BREATHING

Breathing is the first act of life, and the last. Our very life
depends on it. Since we cannot live without breathing, it is
tragically deplorable to contemplate the millions and millions
who have never mastered the art of correct breathing.
Joseph Pilates, *Return to Life through Contrology*

We know breathing is important; without oxygen, we cannot
survive. However, since we don't move our bodies as much
as we should, we don't breathe as much as we should. Your
body emulates what your mind feels, and when your body is
tight and tired, your mind is tight and tired. Most of us do
not think about breathing; it's an automatic thing we do in
order to stay alive. However, breathing is something we can
consciously take over; it does not have to be automatic, and
one of the most powerful things you can do for your health is
to learn how to control your breathing.

Let's take a closer look at the link between our bodies
and our minds. When you have been nervous, have you ever
felt your heart race? The thoughts in your mind caused a
physiological response in your body that automatically raises
your heart rate without your conscious involvement. What
about when you're anxious? Do you ever feel your stomach

go flip-flop a few times? Once again, your body is telling you what your mind is feeling.

Breathing for Energy

Did you know that proper breathing can increase your energy throughout the day? Breathing deeply and more effectively can increase blood flow throughout the body, therefore giving all your muscles and organs more energy.

In theory, if our mind can control our body, then we can use our bodies to control the mind. We can use our mind to tell the body to breathe, which, in turn, gets the mind to relax. Deep circulatory breathing can help to calm the mind and reduce stress. Almost every stress-reduction health plan involves some sort of breathing regimen. Beyond the simple task of oxygenating the blood, breathing can give you a sense of peace and control. You know what the best thing about breathing properly is? It's free, and doesn't take up any more time in your day.

Breathing for Immunity

Did you know that breathing properly can help improve your immune system? The circulation of energy can help regenerate tissue, assist with healing and speed up the recovery process.

How to Breathe

There are a variety of methods and opinions on how to breathe, and each kind of breath has a different purpose. You breathe differently when you are at your computer and when you are meditating, or when you are exercising intensely. The essence of it all is that you must breathe. We will talk more specifically about the kind of breath that helps you excel in a Pilates routine.

There are many muscles in the body involved in the breath cycle; the primary muscles are the diaphragm, which is located in the bottom part of your ribcage, and the intercostal muscles, which are located within the ribcage, between each rib. Some secondary muscles are in the neck region, such as the sternocleidomastoid and the scalenes. All together, these muscles work to bring in as much oxygen as possible, as well as expel the air out of the lungs.

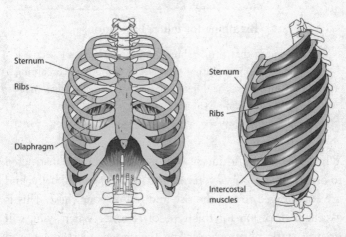

Breathing for Better Skin

Did you know that breathing more effectively can give you better skin? Breathing = blood flow = good circulation = a healthy glow!

Our sedentary lifestyle, combined with improper posture, often causes us to breathe incorrectly. People tend to overuse the upper respiratory muscles, when these are supposed to be secondary to the muscles in the ribcage. As a result, some people experience chronic neck tension. Since these upper respiratory muscles were not meant to do the primary work when breathing, the breath is shallow and ineffective. It takes mental focus and concentration to relearn the proper breath pattern that works well in the variety of circumstances you experience. It's important to relearn how to breathe into the thoracic cavity, where the ribcage is located, instead of your neck.

Breathing for Injury Prevention

Did you know that proper breathing mechanics can decrease your chance of injury during exercise? If you are not breathing correctly during a difficult exercise, the spine and pelvis remain unsupported and can be subject to injury.

When meditating or during yoga practice, you are instructed to breathe as deeply as you can into the ribcage and belly, and are encouraged to feel the rise and fall of your chest. This is excellent direction for this type of routine. When lying still or in a static posture, releasing the chest and stomach and allowing air to fully gather in your lungs is a wonderful way to increase circulation and air in your body. This is also an incredible solution for stress. Focused breathing can reduce stress symptoms almost immediately. When our body is in a state of stress, we tend to tighten up, and our breath becomes shallow.

> **Breathing for Digestion**
>
> Did you know that good breathing can improve digestion? The movement of the diaphragm can massage the internal organs and help in the digestive process.

Breathing for Pilates

In Chapter 8, we will outline a variety of Pilates-based exercises. Keep in mind that when you are performing difficult Pilates exercises, you are required to use a different kind of breath. Instead of releasing all the muscles in the abdominal region, we ask that you continue to maintain a contraction in the transversus abdominis. Remember, the transversus abdominis wraps around your waist and provides a basis for support in the spine. Instead of releasing your belly, we actually want you to keep it engaged throughout your breath pattern. This means that you need to feel your belly muscle pull into the spine and stay there, while you continue to breathe deeply in order to deliver oxygen to the muscles. If you are breathing this way and contracting your belly muscles nice and tight, you might ask, 'So where does the air go?' Well, the air still fills your lungs, though not as effectively as a belly breath. Instead, the emphasis is to breathe into the ribcage and intercostals. We want to see the belly remain as still as possible, and instead watch the ribcage expand out to the sides. While teaching Pilates, a good instructor might call this 'breathing laterally'.

Let's try it together:

Sit on a chair or ball facing a mirror. Hold your waist just below your ribs so that your thumbs are on the back part of your ribs and your index finger on the front part of the lowest rib.

Relax your shoulders and close your eyes. Take a deep breath in, and try to expand the air into your hands, laterally (to the sides). Exhale and feel the air release as your index fingers come back towards each other. Continue for a few more breaths with your eyes closed before you open them and watch the movement of your ribs in the mirror. With your eyes open, take a peek at your belly. Is it releasing forward and creating a pooch in the belly region? If so, close your eyes, contract your abdominals by pulling them into the spine, and try again. Feel the breath move into the index finger and thumb.

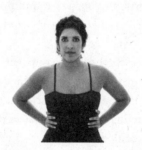

You can also perform this practice lying down. This time, have your hands down by your sides with your knees bent and your feet flat on the floor (for comfort in the lower back). Keep your eyes open and look down your chest towards your belly. On the inhalation, keep the belly from rising up, and instead, feel the breath move into the sides of your arms and into the floor. Then, on the exhalation, watch your belly sink deeper into your spine and the ribs close back up into their starting position.

It takes a long time to learn ribcage breathing in a Pilates practice. There is already so much to think about in a particular exercise that breathing often comes last on the list of priorities. However, as you progress in your routine, you will be able to find more focus on the breath and learn to keep the belly contracted and engaged throughout each exercise.

Breathing for a Younger Look

Did you know that learning how to breathe properly can make you look younger and slimmer? The increase in blood flow can help reduce the signs of ageing on the skin. Learning how to breathe through the ribcage can tone the muscles in the midsection and make your waistline look slimmer.

Nose versus Mouth Breathing

There are varying opinions on the benefits of breathing through the mouth versus through the nose. Pilates emphasizes inhalation through the nose and exhalation through the mouth. Yoga and meditation practitioners ask that you only breathe in and out through the nose. Nose breathing is technically a better way of breathing on the inhalation portion of the exercise. Inhaling through the nose uses the sinuses as a way to filter the air. Exhalation through the mouth is preferred in the Pilates repertoire because it can help activate a deep abdominal contraction, since you can expend more air in a single mouth breath.

There are even a few varying ways to exhale through the mouth. Some encourage a 'ha' sound, with the lips slightly open. Others, such as the first-generation Pilates teacher Ron Fletcher, insisted on a very sharp 'shhhh' sound, with the mouth in an 'o' shape.

For the purposes of the exercises in this book, we encourage you to find a pattern that works for you. Ribcage breathing is a must for spinal support and abdominal strength, so spend some time working on mastering this style of breathing. However, the exhalation component of your breath can be your choice. Be sure to breathe in through the nose every time, but choose what works better for you:

1. Exhale through the nose (yoga inspired).
2. Exhale with 'shhh' (Ron Fletcher inspired).
3. Exhale with 'ha' (inspired by other Pilates practitioners).

Try different options and find what feels more comfortable, then stick with it.

When your Pilates practice is over and you have decided to embark on meditation, allow the belly to let go and feel the air fully fill your lungs. The juxtaposition of the abdominal contraction, followed by a breath pattern with an abdominal release, is a sign that you have just learnt how to control your breath in various ways. This is a form of control over your body that will give you one more tool on the quest for total health.

Coming Up Next

You've learnt the concept of breathing laterally, and finally have some physical homework you can start to work on. Try breathing in front of the mirror every morning and evening immediately after brushing your teeth. As your breathing becomes more controlled, your ability to perform the exercises in Chapter 8 will become greatly enhanced.

Next, we will address the issue that stops most people from achieving any fitness goal they might have: fear. What are you scared of? There are many possibilities and we want to spend some time on this topic to help you gain a deeper understanding of yourself and how you can achieve all the fitness goals you dream of. Don't skip this next one: much like breathing is necessary for life, self-analysis and awareness are necessary for a successful life.

HOW FEAR CAN SHAPE YOU

Self-confidence, poise, consciousness of possessing the power to accomplish our desires, with renewed lively interest in life are the natural results of the practice of Contrology.

Joseph Pilates, *Return to Life through Contrology*

You might be tempted to skip this chapter. Fear? What does fear have to do with achieving the body of my dreams? In one word: everything.

We can tell you what to eat, how to walk and what exercises to do, but unless you are capable of looking inside yourself and understanding how your brain is wired, your chances of successfully implementing the theories in this book will fall short. The emotions you experience play a large role in the way you think. The way you think influences the decisions you make. The decisions you make define the success you will achieve. So we urge you not to skip this chapter, because in the next few pages lie a few secrets that will help you reframe your mind to successfully improve your body.

Have you ever set a goal for yourself and, after a week, discovered that you've lost your motivation? Maybe you woke up one morning and *swore* to yourself that you would drink more water that day, and by 2.00 p.m. you realized you hadn't had a drop of water since 8.00 a.m.? Or perhaps you spent a week working hard to lose a kilo, and, when you had only lost half a kilo, you decided it wasn't worth it and ate that cookie for dinner. Even clients who hire personal trainers to remind them what they need to do will fall prey to 'forgetting' what they set out to accomplish. The trainer can yell at you and berate you, or they can hug and support you, but unless you know how to accomplish change within yourself, their efforts are futile.

What happens when you make a commitment to the people you love, and you break that commitment? If your mother asked you to be at her home at 5.00 p.m., would you be there? If your daughter asked you to help her with her homework after school, would you do it? If your wife asked you to help organize the living room over the weekend, would you oblige? We venture to say that the answer to these questions is probably 'yes'. What happens when you tell yourself you will do your exercises every day at 3.00 p.m.? Shouldn't that commitment to yourself be just as important as those that you make to the people you love? The commitments to our own desire to change are greatly influenced by what happens inside our own head.

Conscious versus Subconscious

Let's first talk about the mind. First, and ever-present, is the conscious mind. This is the part of your mind that is reading this book. It's what is omnipresent in your logical thoughts. The conscious mind tells you what you want to eat, it tells you to lift that dumb-bell and it will ask you to drink water. It's what you know and think, and stores all the thoughts within your awareness. When you decide to lie down and do some deep breathing, you do this with your conscious mind.

Second, and more mysterious, is the subconscious mind. This is where you house the involuntary actions that you don't think about, such as blinking and swallowing. When your heart rate rises as a result of being nervous or scared, your subconscious mind is at work. This is also where your emotions live, and often, these emotions are a result of your past experiences. The subconscious mind is the part of you that you have little control over; the part where your instincts lie; the part where your deepest fears reside. It's extremely influential over the rest of your mind, yet you have little control over it. Sometimes, parts of the subconscious reveal themselves in the form of dreams or Freudian slips. Have you ever accidently called your current boyfriend by your ex-boyfriend's name? That is a Freudian slip. This is the subconscious mind at work. Perhaps your mind is telling you that you haven't quite yet moved on from that ex-boyfriend.

Fear versus Love

Now that we understand the mind a little more, let's talk about emotions. There are only two basic emotions in life: love and fear. In love, we are happy. We are peaceful. We are gracious and giving. In fear, we can be aggressive, angry, resentful and hurtful. In fear, we aim to protect ourselves; we do everything in our power not to get hurt. It's a survival instinct that often resides in our subconscious. You may be consciously aware of some fears, such as your fear of spiders or snakes. There are other types of fear, such as fear of failure or of abandonment. These types of fear reside in our subconscious and can influence the choices we make without really knowing or understanding them.

We would like to give you an example that speaks of how the fears in the subconscious can influence your actions. This example uses the mind of a child and, because the mind of a child is pure, it is the perfect place to see how these theories meet reality.

We know a mother who lovingly adopted a child from an orphanage. This child was over a year old when she found her way to her new mother. In that year, she had been abandoned and neglected. This child did not receive the care that most children from loving homes receive from birth. She would cry for help and not receive a response. She would compete with other children for food and she was not accustomed to being hugged and cared for. For the first few years that this child was with her adoptive mother, she struggled to accept her. She hit her, she pulled her hair and she screamed for hours on end when she didn't get her way. If the mom didn't know better, she could have reprimanded the child for misbehaving, but luckily, the mom did know better. The child would hug her mother and cling to her, then push her away and defy her. This child was torn by the fears in her subconscious. She wanted her mommy, but lived in a constant state of fear of losing her.

As this child got older and learnt to speak, her fears became clearer to her mother. One day when the mom left her side to run an errand, the child's heart started to race. She began to sweat. She repeated to herself, 'I will never see my mommy again. I will never see my mommy again.' When the mom returned, the child hugged her and clung to her. The child's experiences as a young baby, being abandoned and neglected, left an imprint that influenced her actions for years to come. The child could not remember her first year in her orphanage. But the impact of the emotions housed themselves deep in her subconscious. One hopes, in time, this child's story of abandonment and neglect will dissipate. Instead, she will replace her fears with the years of love, attention and caring; eventually unconditional love will take over, and conquer all fear.

If you've picked up this book with the intention of changing your body, you must first address your mind. What fears might be lodged so deeply in your subconscious mind that they prevent you from making changes? What is your story? Here are some ideas.

Fear of Change

You grew up being told you were too slim, or too chubby. You were always picked last for the cricket team since you were not very good at it. Or, perhaps, you would eat anything you wanted and would never gain weight. Once these ideas are lodged in your brain, they stay there, often in the subconscious. You grow older, your metabolism starts to slow down, and suddenly your body gains kilos even though your diet hasn't changed. Or, maybe you've never been great at athletics but you have decided that it is time to start an exercise routine. Easy, right? Just follow the exercises in this book, and you will be in the best shape of your life.

This seems easy but if you've ever tried to change, the road is often paved with ups and downs, and twists and turns. Your subconscious is telling you one thing: change is scary. It tells you that 'you are who you are' and it's safer to stay the same. Deep inside your mind, it's saying that eating healthy is going to be scary because it's hard to do. It's also telling you that exercise is new, therefore, it's scary. It's telling you that you are fine just the way you are, the way you have always been. Your conscious mind wants to change, but your subconscious fears start putting obstacles in your path. You rationalize in your conscious mind that it's okay to skip your workout since your daughter needed you to help with her homework. Or, you claim you didn't have the time, since your hair-and-nail appointment was a priority.

The fear of change is powerful because it directly affects our self-perception. If we grew up with a parent who constantly bugged us about being overweight, then these self-perceptions may be deep-seated . You look in the mirror, and all you see is fat. Even if you've lost weight, it still might be all you see. Despite the fact that you have changed on the outside, you may not see the changes on the inside. Sure, our parents are not to blame as they do the best they can in raising us. However, the words you hear growing up can make a lasting impression on who you are, and whether you are capable of undergoing an emotional change with ease.

Overcoming the Fear of Change

The first step on the path to change is to create awareness about the things that might get in your way. If you recognize and acknowledge your fears, they become easier to see and fight. With fear of change, it's important to identify what it is you want to be versus what you think your past is creating. For example, let's say you have always been overweight, and it is your goal to become slim. It is important to start seeing yourself as a slim and lean person even before you lose the weight. Positive affirmations are an excellent way to achieve this. Affirmations are words and phrases to help influence your thoughts. Affirmations and positive thinking are key components to effect change. If you're in a constant state of negativity ('I will never lose weight'), then chances are you will never lose weight. A more powerful thought would be to say, 'I am lean.' 'I am size small.' 'I am a skinny person.' These are examples of words and phrases to say to yourself in order to eventually achieve what you want to become. If the goal is to learn to take Pilates, but you've never been flexible, this obstacle can block you from even attempting your first exercise. 'I am limber.' 'I am powerful and flexible.' 'I embrace a Pilates body.'

Fear of Failure

Failure is an ugly word. With failure comes judgement and shame . . . and fear. Once again, some fears are obvious and lodged in the conscious mind: 'I'm scared of doing that exercise because it looks like I may fall off the machine.' Other fears are so deeply entrenched in your subconscious that you are unaware of them and you innocently embark on your weight-loss journey.

Let's assume you grew up rather active and played sports. There were wins and there were defeats. You learnt that

Flabby Tummy?

I (Yasmin) have spent the greater part of my life focused on my fitness. I exercise regularly. I eat immaculately, and am proud of what I have accomplished with my body and my career. Except, when I look in the mirror, I always see a flabby tummy. How can I, one of India's premier fitness trainers, have a flabby tummy? In reality, it's not true. I have a trim midsection that clients admire and aim to achieve. But growing up, I was always told that my stomach bulged out, and therefore this idea has lodged into my subconscious and my conscious brain. I always feared that I would never get rid of this belly. In my case, I am addicted to facing my fears. Instead of letting this rule me and push me away from fitness, it fuelled me to search for ways to solve this problem. The result is my career in Pilates. However, we are all human, and I still work to overcome the visual that I have of myself with a flabby tummy. I aim to look in the mirror and see what I know I am: fit, lean and powerful in my centre.

one is way more appealing than the other. Defeat and failure are not nearly as fun as being successful and winning. So you worked hard and you practised, you did your cross-training, you worked with the best coach and you prepared for the game the best way you knew. Regardless of your efforts, you still lost. The defeat is too devastating, and you think 'maybe it's safer to not play at all'. Further, the subconscious mind might process the emotions from your devastating loss into an internal attitude of 'I'm no good at this no matter how hard I try.'

Perhaps your story is not even that obvious. Let's say athletics was not your thing. Instead, you were an artist.

You learnt early on that you were excellent at art, and the praise and support you received every time you produced an excellent painting felt so good that you stuck with it. You never attempted anything outside your comfort zone. Why? Because you were content to stay with what you knew. Subconsciously, you were protecting yourself. Failure was not possible if you stuck with what you knew.

So now you're in your thirties or forties and it's time to take your health seriously. You've never really paid much attention to it, but your conscious mind doesn't like what it sees in the mirror, so it's time to concentrate on losing some weight. You read this book. You go shopping for healthy food, and perhaps you even join the gym. But the underlying voice in your subconscious starts to speak up. You spend a few days making a salad, then, before you know it, the pizza they always serve at lunch starts to call your name again. Your conscious mind receives the input from the subconscious mind. So, your conscious mind rationalizes it: 'Oh, it's just one day. It won't kill me.' Boom! Motivation lost.

Overcoming the Fear of Failure

Once again, acknowledgement of fears is paramount to success. Simply by reading this chapter and examining what might be blocking your way, you are taking steps forward. When it comes to fear of failure, it's important to set yourself up for success right from the beginning. Don't set unrealistic goals: stick with something you can accomplish and achieve success in. If you know you want to lose 20 kilos, start by looking to lose 5 kilos first. Cross that accomplishment off your list, overcome your fear of failure and move on to the next goal. If you want to become a Pilates expert, start with mastering the first two exercises in Chapter 8. Feel successful, and then move on.

Fear of failure surfaces daily, at times, without attracting much attention. We sabotage our diet because we're afraid we won't be able to sustain it. We avoid taking the aerobics class because we are afraid we won't be able to keep up. So, with these particular fears, visualization techniques can be quite successful. Visualize your day from the beginning to end and take note where you might be subject to your fears. Visualize yourself in class, performing the exercises well. Close your eyes and visualize what it must feel like to feel proud of the food you selected to eat. Visualization of success will make you far more likely to achieve it.

Techniques for Conquering Fear

There are thousands of programmes out there that will attempt to help you reprogramme your subconscious. There are thousands of coaches and motivational speakers who litter the Internet telling you it's easy to change how you think. These methods, however, give the false impression that these people and external sources can facilitate change. The reality is, only you can fix yourself. Be aware; listen to your body and its reaction to your emotions. Does the idea of exercising daily make your palms sweaty? Does looking at a healthy salad make your stomach turn over? If you're lucky enough to get these obvious signals from your body, then listen to them and take notice.

Running Marathons

I (Zeena) participated in many extracurricular activities as a young child. Soccer, softball, dance and gymnastics were all things that I tried. Sports ended up not suiting me, and instead, I gravitated towards dance and cheerleading. As an adult, when I found myself wanting to lose some kilos, it was completely foreign to me since the only real exercise I had done in my life was dance. Running? Lifting weights? Playing volleyball? None of it sounded like anything 'Zeena' could do. 'Zeena' was a graceful dancer who didn't do anything too strenuous. At least, this was the story in my head.

Luckily, I heard of a programme that helped you train for a marathon. The idea of running 26.2 miles was overwhelming, but the programme broke it down for you into smaller, digestible sections. You would train 3–4 miles a few times a week (I could do that) and would add only one extra mile to your run every Saturday. The weekly goals were achievable. If I was capable of running 8 miles one Saturday, why couldn't I run nine the next? Of course, I could, and I did. And I even beat my target time on the day of the race, by 35 seconds. Fear of failure? Sure. Did I choose a plan with realistic goals that set me up for success? Absolutely.

Meditation

Much like exercising your body, you need to spend time exercising your mind. We've discussed overcoming particular fears by using positive affirmations and visualizations. Both affirmations and visualizations can be practised with daily meditation. Meditation is the best and easiest way to spend quality time looking inward. Never meditated before? With the advent of technology, shutting down the outside world has become easier. It's now possible for you to put earphones into your ears in the middle of a crowded room, play some meditation music from one of the hundreds of apps, and disappear into yourself.

Let's look into the science behind meditation. The brain gives off waves, and there are four different levels of brainwaves:

1) Beta (14–40 Hz): This is when you are in a full state of consciousness.
2) Alpha (7.5–14 Hz): This is when you begin to relax more, and enter a state closer to your subconscious. You are able to tap into your intuition better in this state.
3) Theta (4–7.5 Hz): This is when you aim to be in a state of meditation. You are fully relaxed and sometimes feel like you are floating.
4) Delta (0.5–4 Hz): This is when you are asleep.

The goal of meditation is to relax and get to the alpha or theta levels within your brain, tap into your intuition and create awareness of your subconscious beliefs. If you feel like you are floating but still have a conscious awareness of where you are and feel entirely relaxed, chances are you have achieved this level of brainwaves. Tapping into this level of your brain will give you the awareness you need to effect change. Clarity can be found and mental focus can be regained.

If you find it impossible to sit still and find this level of relaxation, don't be alarmed. You are not alone! There are different meditation guides that can assist you in this process. You can listen to their words, and focus on breathing and relaxation techniques. Often, the proper music can help to influence and slow down your brainwaves. With these guided meditations come affirmations and visualizations that can help you with your particular issues.

Know Your Stories

Even more detrimental to factors creating positive changes are the 'stories' that you create about yourself that clearly define your limitations. A client might say in their first session, 'I hurt my knee, so I will never be able to run again.' Upon further investigation, we find out that the knee injury actually happened when the client was 17 years old, which was over 20 years ago. Surprised that a 20-year-old injury was still causing daily pain, we ask the client to rate the pain on a scale of one to ten. The client responds that they are not currently in pain, but they 'know' that they will be if they try to run. This obstacle is as clear as day; the story from their past experience is not only locked deeply in their subconscious mind, it's permeated into their consciousness. How do they 'know' that their knee will hurt forever? Fear of change and fear of failure are both at work here. Sure, knee pain may be their history, but it's their own mind that has determined that this pain will be there forever. The reality is, with proper alignment, great posture and strong muscles, a 20-year-old injury should not be causing pain and often can be easily resolved.

Affirmations

When the stories you create for yourself are this obvious, affirmations can be of great assistance. Here is an idea that might help you. Post some affirmations on your window and say them to yourself when you wake up. Repeat them in your daily meditation. Write them down in your journal at night. Even better, repeat them during your daily workout!

Here are some basic affirmations to help you on the quest towards change:

I am healthy, I am fit.
I choose to be strong.
I honour my body with good eating.
The weight will fall off my body.
I release my past and embrace my future.
I am in alignment in body and mind.
I know I can and I will.
I will work hard and succeed.
Positivity leaves no place for negative thoughts.

Coming Up Next

You've learnt a bit about how the mind works, and you understand the importance of self-awareness and affirmations. You are now aware of your emotions and your fears, and how these can affect long-term change. Now it's time to take a closer look at how emotions play a part in your body alignment, mechanics and, more importantly, how body alignment affects how you look. Posture and exercise can directly affect how you feel. How you feel can affect how you walk, sit and stand. Much like Joseph Pilates asked you to concentrate on your body, we will spend a few more pages dedicated to helping you make a deeper connection to this mind–body awareness.

SHAPING YOUR EMOTIONS

*Logically, man should develop his physical condition
simultaneously with the development of his mind—neither
should be sacrificed at the expense of the other; otherwise
'Balance of Body and Mind' is not attainable, and this very
lack of harmony between man's physical and mental health,
is primarily responsible for man's unfortunate physical and
mental condition today.*

Joseph Pilates, *Your Health*

Earlier, we explained the biomechanics that cause your shoulders to round and your spine to lose its alignment. We also explained which muscles get tight and which ones get weak. These are all physical descriptions of what happens to the body when it starts to lose alignment. But, as we just explained, there is a mind–body connection; so how do our minds and our emotions play into this?

Have you ever gone on stage to recite a prayer, perform a dance or make a speech, and found yourself sweating profusely? Maybe your hands were shaking and your stomach was doing somersaults? Maybe you can't sleep the night before a big party that you've been planning for months? These symptoms are your body's way of processing emotion. Fear, stress, nervous energy and excitement are all emotions. Your brain feels these emotions and provides you with physical manifestations of them. The same thing happens with your body's posture.

In 2010, there was some research conducted and published on behalf of the Association for Psychological Science by Dana R. Carney, Amy J.C. Cuddy and Andy J. Yap. We found their findings incredibly fascinating, and applicable to our argument for the link between posture and emotions. Specifically, the researchers in this study aimed to test the link between body postures and two hormones: cortisol and testosterone.

Testosterone is closely linked with dominance and power. The more you have, the more powerful you feel. Testosterone increases in anticipation of a challenge, and decreases upon defeat. Cortisol is the hormone linked to stress. When your stress level goes up, your body creates more cortisol as a way to help you manage the stress. However, since increased cortisol levels can weaken the immune system, long-term, chronically elevated cortisol levels are not good for your body, and can result in an assortment of physiological issues. Cortisol has an inverse relationship to testosterone; that is to say that when one goes up, the other comes down. Powerful people often have lower cortisol levels and higher testosterone levels. People who feel powerless have the opposite: higher cortisol and lower testosterone.

Carney, Cuddy and Yap did some testing on the impact of 'power poses' and how they can affect the way you feel. They asked participants to either hold a 'high-power pose' or a 'low-power pose' for two minutes. High-power poses involved standing with the chest lifted and arms open, and the posture involved taking up a lot of space. Low-power poses were much smaller in scale—the shoulders were hunched and, perhaps, the arms crossed. After holding the postures for two minutes, the participants took a saliva test for testosterone and cortisol. In addition, the researchers tested the participants' desire and/or ability to take risks by asking them if they wanted to gamble some money. Participants could choose whether they wanted to gamble two dollars to possibly make four dollars, or walk away with their money in hand.

The results confirmed the link between high-power poses, lower cortisol levels (less stress) and higher testosterone (more power). The saliva test showed that testosterone went up and cortisol went down after a participant held the high-power pose for 2 minutes. For the low-power-pose participants, the saliva test confirmed that their testosterone had dropped and their cortisol had increased. When it came to gambling, the high-power posers elected to gamble 86 per cent of the time, over the lower-power posers who decided to gamble only 60 per cent of the time. So there you have it. If posture has a direct effect on your hormones, and hormones have a direct effect on your emotions, then the link is clear. Improve your posture, and your mind will follow.

In addition, how you feel on the inside provides a link to how you are perceived on the outside. Your first and last impressions are often non-verbal. Therefore, your posture can exhibit certain emotions to the people you are interacting with. Let's take a look at each individual postural deviation. From there, we will discuss the different ways someone might be perceived from the outside, or the emotion that they might feel on the inside.

Posture	Internal Emotions	Perception to Others
Hunchback	Fatigue Lack of energy	Lack of confidence Emotionally protected
Flat back	Fatigue Lack of energy Shame	Appears shorter and wider Lack of confidence Embarrassment
Arched back	Not feeling 'centred' Vulnerable	Overconfident Not looking 'centred'

Hunchback Posture

This is the most common posture in modern society, and it's the most obvious to see. If you take a look at the ageing population, you will notice that a majority of people over the age of sixty have a certain degree of hunchback. Many have this posture to such an extreme that they lose multiple inches of their frame. Have you ever heard that Pilates can make you taller? If you think about this, it's rather silly because without the use of growth hormone steroids, it's impossible to truly grow taller. However, since a majority of the population struggles with some degree of hunchback posture, fixing it can have the appearance of looking taller since you are standing up straighter.

What is the most common emotion relevant to the ageing population? Fatigue. What happens to the muscles in your back when they are not strong enough to hold up your frame? They are fatigued. Hunchback posture, technically known as kyphosis, can otherwise be described as the'fatigue' posture. In an older person, this posture is expected. However, more and more, this is becoming a popular ailment among younger generations due to the body positioning associated with constant texting and computer work. This younger population is not generally fatigued (as some sixty-year-olds might be), instead, their back muscles have atrophied and can no longer hold their body up in the correct position.

Hunchback posture can give the appearance of lack of energy. Someone's energy can make a lasting (first) impression. Good posture is as important as eye contact, and as memorable as a handshake. Without proper energy, someone might be overlooked for their dream job, or be rejected by a possible love interest.

Standing with your shoulders forward can also give the impression of being emotionally 'protected'. What are you protecting? In this posture, the most important organ in our body is shielded: the heart. Instead of your chest being lifted and open, it's dropped and closed. Worse, if this posture is accompanied by neck or back pain, then this 'closed' posture drives these emotions to an even deeper level. Pain creates a short circuit of energy within the body.

In addition to the emotions that are perceived, standing with a hunchback makes you look shorter, shortens your waistline and pooches your stomach. Again, this speaks to someone's perceived confidence and energy.

Flat-Back Posture

Flat-back posture is when the lower spine is missing the curve, and the appearance of the butt is wide and flat. The tail bone, the bony landmark that should be pointing directly down, is actually tucked underneath the body. A flat back is almost always accompanied by the hunchback posture, and exhibits many of the same signs, internally and externally. By adding the lower spine into the equation, it just magnifies the intensity of the emotions, as well as the possible accompanying pain.

As mentioned above, this posture could be indicative of ageing and fatigue, but again, this posture has become popular with people who sit and hunch forward for a living. Most clients sit at a desk, looking straight ahead with their head jutted forward, their whole spine rounded and their tail tucked beneath them on their chair. No matter how interesting or intense the content on their computer screen might be, their body only exhibits and expends a very small amount of energy.

Have you ever seen a dog when he has been bad and is hiding his tail underneath him? This is the best way to articulate what is going on when someone has a flat back and hunchback combined. Their tail is literally tucked underneath them. The heart is closed off from both ends of their spine. They look shorter, less confident and more protected. It may even seem to the outside world that they are giving off an air of shame or embarrassment. Did the posture create the shame, or did a sense of shame define the posture? Regardless of the order and the reasoning, this combined posture is indicative of the most desperate and depressing of emotional states.

Arched Back

Arched back, or lordotic posture, is when the butt protrudes out in an exaggerated fashion and the lower back has an excessive curve. People with arched-back posture usually have tight hip flexors and weak abdominals. The connection to their core is often severed and they have limited ability to engage their abdominals. Pilates can be extremely challenging for people in this particular demographic.

Bad-Dog Posture

I (Zeena) recently had a client who came to me in extreme back pain, and was frustrated with her inability to work out. She had been a high-intensity athlete in the past, and her inability to continue these workouts was affecting her immensely. At first glance, I was sure she wouldn't buy sessions from me. She was quiet, barely made eye contact and didn't seem to want to be standing in my studio. I knew her problem right away: she had extreme hunchback and flat-back posture. Looking back, my perception of her then was so negative: she seemed uninterested and had no confidence in herself. I was surprised when she signed up for the sessions! We reviewed some stretches and exercises for her to do and started working on implementing a change in her posture. Over time, her pain subsided and she increased her workout intensity. Then one day, I walked in, saw her and asked: 'Did you change your hairstyle?' 'No,' she said, but then, I realized the real reason she looked different. She was standing taller and was not in pain any more. She talked more, smiled sometimes and even cracked a joke or two. It was like we had a whole new client. The power of posture is real.

Often, arched-back posture is interesting in that the emotion conveyed is that of extreme confidence. Models and actors will place their bodies, inadvertently, in an arched-back position as a way to lift their chest tall and proud. If they lift their upper body and flare their ribs out, and the abdominals are not strong enough to support this movement, the lower spine will compensate by swaying backwards. This display of confidence is wonderful. If you are proud of your butt and want to show it off, we encourage this! However, this is only a positive experience if it's not accompanied by the possible pain associated with arched-back issues. Abdominal strength is the key.

Another interesting experience we have encountered with those who have an arched back posture is the loss of connection to their core. Women who have had C-section births can sometimes fall into this category. The core is the centre of the body. It's where movement begins. Without a connection to this centre, there is a strong possibility of chronic back pain in the lumbar spine. Clients with arched backs, weak abdominals and lower back pain usually have no understanding of the misalignment in their spine. They are confused when we explain that their lower back is taking far more stress than it can handle. Their awareness is limited and their sense of centre is off.

It's an interesting group to teach, as they must relearn how to engage their abdominals, as well as their pelvic floor. The pelvic-floor muscles are the muscles in the base of the spine that control the functions of urination and bowel movements. These muscles are critical to the support of the spine and the feeling of being centred. Every Pilates exercise should be accompanied by a pelvic-floor contraction so as to support the spine within the movement. If you are in an arched-back posture, then the likelihood is high that you will have a harder time contracting your pelvic floor. Without strong abdominal muscles and without pelvic floor awareness, the overall 'centre' of the body is simply missing. How do you feel when you don't feel centred? We venture to guess that you might feel out of control, lost or even vulnerable.

Recovering from Cancer

I (Yasmin) had someone very dear to me go through a fight with cancer. His treatment plan involved rigorous bouts of chemotherapy, which would wipe him out and make it difficult to do anything for ten days after his treatment. However, after the 10-day period would pass, he was done with feeling 'unwell'. He is a person who usually always had a good attitude, but lying in bed and feeling rounded in his body and posture made things morbid. He decided to take control of his body instead of allowing the disease to get the better of him. So he walked into my Pilates studio and decided to get stronger. He took it slowly, as his body would not allow him to push himself, but he worked towards his goal. In the process, he opened up his spine, he moved with control, he changed his hunchback posture he had gained by lying in bed. The result was a more confident position, which also enhanced his positive attitude. He continued his commitment to doing Pilates as often as he could in between his chemotherapy appointments. He now has more control and power over his body and his disease.

Coming Up Next

You now understand a bit more about how emotions can affect the body. You now see and understand the value of the mind–body connection. Now it's time to get down to the nitty-gritty. Next, you will finally learn how to work your body properly. You will learn how to engage your centre, how to warm up your spine and what exercises to select to help you with your particular posture misalignment. You will be given a chance to create your own custom workout that you can do daily, to help you achieve your fitness goals.

EXERCISES TO SCULPT AND SHAPE

*Concentrate on the correct movements EACH TIME
YOU EXERCISE, lest you do them improperly and
thus lose all the vital benefits of their value. Correctly
executed and mastered to the point of subconscious
reaction, these exercises will reflect grace and balance in
your routine activities.*
Joseph Pilates, *Return to Life through Contrology*

It's time to get down to the real business of Pilates: the exercises.

You can eat very well, drink enough water and do cardio every day, but unless you do weight-bearing exercise, it will be difficult to create a well-sculpted body. The fat in your body will burn off with proper nutrition and cardio, but building some amount of muscle is necessary to sculpt a well-shaped figure. The beauty of the routine you will read about in this chapter is that all it takes is you and a mat.

We will begin by outlining some basic rules for performing Pilates. Each routine will begin with two warm-up exercises and one cool-down exercise. Each of the warm-up and cool-down exercises can be performed by anyone, regardless of their postural alignment.

After the warm-up exercises, you will see the exercises divided into three groups. You will choose two out of the three groups, thereby creating a comprehensive workout. Everyone should perform the exercises for hunchback (the only upper-body postural issue), and then choose from among the two lower-body groups, depending on what works best for them (flat back or arched back).

Engaging Your TVA

As you may remember, in Chapter 2, we discussed the important transversus abdominus muscle, which wraps around your spine. This is a very important muscle to pay attention to when performing Pilates exercises. Think of it as a weight belt—the TVA wraps around the pelvis and keeps it in place. This added stability aids in preventing injuries to the hips and spine. Without proper contraction of the TVA, the belly will protrude outward and can actually increase the likelihood of injury during a challenging Pilates routine. Let's practise how to engage this muscle properly before we embark on your exercise routine.

Sit up tall in your chair and place both of your hands on top of each other, on top of your stomach. Take a moment to push the belly into your hands and notice what this feels like. Now do the opposite: pull your belly away from your hands and suck it in towards your spine. Again, notice how this feels. Practise this 2 more times. Push out and then pull in.

Then, shift to the front of your chair. Sit tall on your sitz bones (as mentioned earlier, these are the bones in your bottom), make sure you are not slouching and do not have your tail bone tucked under you. Keep both feet firmly planted on the floor. Lean backwards until you feel your abdominals engage. Now, place your hands on your belly and push out, and then pull in. Do you feel a difference here from the attempts above? Try to keep your belly pulled in, and lean back a little further. Do you feel how keeping your belly muscle pulled in allows you to support yourself much better in the backward-leaning position? This is because you have engaged your TVA.

If you are struggling to feel or engage the TVA, try coughing a few times. Pay attention to what happens in your abdominal area when you cough. The muscle you feel pulling in towards your spine is your TVA.

It's quite easy to engage the TVA while sitting and coughing. However, once you start to perform some of the exercises we give you, you will find that your belly wants to push out rather than pull in. Over time, this pulling manoeuvre will become easier as the muscles become stronger and their endurance increases.

Engaging Your Pelvic Floor

Your pelvic-floor muscles are located in your pubic area, and are often overlooked when it comes to exercise. The main muscles are the levator ani muscles and the coccygeus. They are critical to the stabilization of the spine, and assist in building a strong centre. They can assist in achieving a deeper TVA contraction, and vice versa. For both men and women, the sensation of the pelvic floor contracting is often compared to stopping a stream of urine or halting a bowel movement. We call the muscles around the urethra 'pelvic floor 1', and the muscles around the anus 'pelvic floor 2'. Here is an exercise to help you find and utilize your pelvic floor.

Lie face up on the floor with your knees bent, and your arms down by your side. Like you did in the above exercise, pull your belly muscle in towards your spine and hold it there.

Take a deep breath and allow the belly to rise up to the ceiling, then exhale and pull your belly into your spine while blowing all the air out through your mouth. Now do this again. Inhale and let the belly release; this time, as you pull it down, also attempt to clench the muscles around your urethral area, as if someone has just walked in while you are in the process of using the restroom. Nothing in your body should physically move; it should look to someone on the outside like nothing has happened. Exhale and release.

Finally, take another deep breath in and allow the belly to rise. On the exhale, pull in your belly, engage pelvic floor 1 and, if possible, pelvic floor 2 as well. The sensation should be similar to the feeling you have when you stop midway through your bowel release.

If you feel the external butt muscles clench, and you feel your butt lift off the floor, then you have done this incorrectly. You should be able to engage your pelvic floor 2 muscles without using your actual glute muscles. Release everything, concentrate and try again.

These muscles should be engaged as often as possible in your Pilates practice. The best way to increase the neuromuscular awareness around these muscles is to practise without movement, as described above.

Remembering to Breathe

As we discussed in Chapter 6, breathing is essential to increasing the body's performance; the breath is a very important component of every Pilates exercise. In each exercise in the following list, we will give you guidelines on when to inhale and when to exhale. Remember to make sure that you always inhale through the nose. When exhaling, we give you the option of either breathing out through the nose or through the mouth (see Chapter 4 for more details). The most important part of breathing in Pilates is to make sure you are breathing 'laterally'. This means you keep your TVA pulled in towards your spine, and instead, breathe into the back and sides of your ribcage. This will ensure your abdominal region is supported while performing these challenging exercises.

Why Are We Inhaling through the Nose?

In Chapter 5, we gave you two options with regard to breathing in Pilates: inhaling through the nose and exhaling through the nose or inhaling through the nose and exhaling through the mouth. Either way, inhalation must be done through the nose. This is because the nasal cavity and sinuses are designed to filter the impurities in the air. It is also meant to slow down the breath so that you are not hyperventilating through the mouth. Practise this during the following exercises and be sure to inhale slowly and deeply through your nasal cavity.

Pacing

It's difficult to describe in a book how fast or slow to perform an exercise, but it must be noted that Pilates should be performed much slower than other modes of exercise. Unlike spin or step class, or kick-boxing, a practitioner of

Pilates should move rhythmically and slowly. The faster you go with these exercises, the more you use momentum, while the slower you go, the more you activate your muscles. The goal of this workout is to build more muscle and help you get stronger, stand taller and increase your metabolism. Please do not attempt to move through any inhalation or exhalation portion of an exercise in less than 1 second. The average movement should require 2–4 seconds to perform, unless you are holding a position for an extended period of time. We will indicate if there is a holding position for each exercise. We will also suggest how long to hold a position, and give you long-term goals to strive to accomplish.

Finding a Neutral Pelvis

There are many exercises that must be performed with a neutral pelvis. This means that we want a natural lumbar curve in the spine, which can be hard to find if you are naturally round back or arched back. In Chapter 2, we walked you through an assessment; we asked you to stand and place your hands in a triangle on your pelvis, to help determine your natural pelvis position. When lying on the floor about to perform an exercise, the technique to find a neutral pelvis is the same. Place your hands in a triangle position, with your index fingers touching and your thumbs touching. Place this triangle on your stomach area, with your fingertips touching your pubic bone and your thumbs below your belly button. Lift your head and look down at your hands. Are your fingers on the same level with your thumbs? If so, then you are in neutral position.

Some people believe that lying down with a neutral-pelvis position means that there is always a space between the lower back and the floor. This may not be true once you take into account people's sizes, where they carry their fat and how big the glutes are. It's really better to utilize anatomical landmarks such as the pubic bone and hip bones to determine the positioning of the pelvis.

When Should I Modify or Advance?

You will notice in the exercise descriptions that we have listed a modification and an advanced version. If you have an injury, or are currently in some kind of musculoskeletal pain, then we highly recommend you try the 'modified' version of the exercise to begin with. If it feels easy and pain-free, then you may move on to the primary description of the exercise.

If you can easily perform the exercise as described, then you should most definitely give the advanced version a try. The goal is to find a challenge (shaking muscles, breaking into perspiration) without adding any undue strain to the body. We estimate that if you do your Pilates routine every day, you should be able to move to the advanced version within three months.

Warm Up

Everyone needs a short warm up before performing the Pilates repertoire. The following two exercises are recommended for everyone and should be performed every day before you begin your routine.

Pelvic Curl

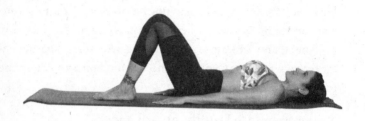

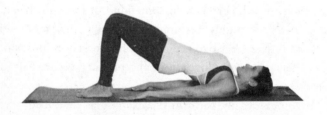

Overall goal: Comprehensive leg and spine warm up.

Postural significance: Strengthens the gluteals and hamstrings. Strengthens the deep intrinsic abdominals. Stretches the hip flexors (applicable to all postures).

Set-up: Lie face up with the knees bent and feet placed flat on the mat. Heels should be a hip-width distance apart. Arms should be by the side with the palms facing down. Pelvis should be in neutral position.

Inhale: Prepare for the movement and hold.

Exhale: Engage the abdominals and curl the pelvis under by pushing the lower back into the mat. Slowly roll the hips up lifting the lower back off the mat first, then the middle back, then the upper back.

Inhale: Prepare for the movement and hold.

Exhale: Slowly roll back down through the spine, placing one vertebra at a time down into the mat. Be sure to end in neutral position.

Notes: Keep the knees in parallel position. Don't let the head or shoulders lift off the mat.

Repetitions: 10.

Modification: For beginners or people with lower back pain, do not lift too high and move through a comfortable range of motion.

Advanced: Bring one leg up off the floor into a tabletop position with the knee over the hip and the lower leg parallel to the mat. Continue the exercise with one leg down and one leg up for 10 repetitions. Then switch legs with one foot on the mat, and the other leg in a tabletop position.

Supine Spine Twist

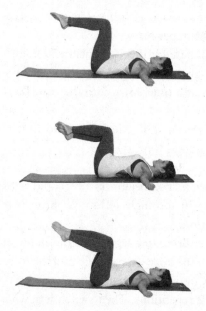

Overall goal: Preparing the spine for rotation.

Postural significance: Strengthens deep intrinsic abdominals and obliques. Strengthens hip flexors. (Applicable for all postures.)

Set-up: Lie face up with the knees in a tabletop position, with the knees directly over the hips and the lower legs parallel to the mat. Place the arms out to the sides in a T position with the palms face down.

Inhale: Lower both legs to one side, keeping the knees glued together. Keep the opposite shoulder down on the mat. If your shoulder raises off the mat, then your legs have gone too far.

Exhale: Engage the abdominals and bring the knees back into the tabletop position.

Inhale: Repeat on the other side.

Exhale: Engage the abdominals and bring the knees back into the tabletop position.

Notes: Don't let the top leg slide down from the bottom leg.

Repetitions: 10 on each side.

Modification: For beginners, keep the feet flat on the floor with the knees together and perform the exercise the same way.

Advanced: After lowering the legs to one side, extend the knees and straighten the legs. Hold this for a breath and then bring the legs back to the centre, and return the knees back to the tabletop position.

Hunchback-Posture Exercises

The following exercises are for clients with the hunchback posture. These are clients who have an excessive rounding-forward of the upper spine. We recommend these exercises to everyone because they are important in counteracting the effects of our modern-day lifestyle, in which we are incessantly texting or hunched over a computer. This posture is most seen in people who sit in front of a computer for a living, or are constantly glued to their phones. (Please see page 34 onwards for a detailed description of all three postural deviations and risk factors.)

Please perform all seven of the exercises given below after you have completed your warm up.

Spine Stretch Forward

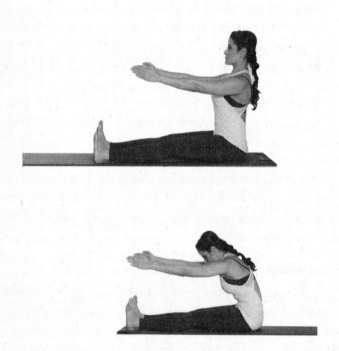

Overall goal: Stretching the spine, strengthening the postural muscles and stretching the hamstrings.

Postural significance: Strengthens back extensors, strengthens deep intrinsic abdominals.

Set-up: Sit with the legs extended slightly wider than hip-width distance. Flex the feet, bringing the toes towards the knees. Sit up tall on the sitz bones. Extend the arms out in front with the palms facing each other.

Inhale: Prepare for the movement and hold.

Exhale: Lower your chin to your chest and start to roll your spine down one vertebra at a time. Stretch the arms over the legs in front of you as if your arms are sliding on a table. Pretend that you are rounding over a small beach ball in front the abdominals.

Inhale: Prepare for the movement and hold.

Exhale: Engage the abdominals and begin to roll the spine back up, one vertebra at a time, until you reach your starting position.

Notes: Make sure the shoulders stay down and away from the ears.

Repetitions: 10.

Modification: For tight hamstrings, bend the knees slightly or sit up on a yoga block to help straighten the legs. You can also perform this exercise up against a wall to feel the articulation of the spine against a flat surface for better results.

Advanced: After rounding forward, lengthen the spine into a flat-back, diagonal position and bring the arms up parallel to the ears. Round forward again and roll up into the starting position.

Side Bend

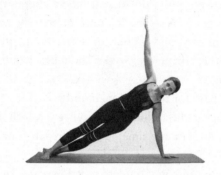

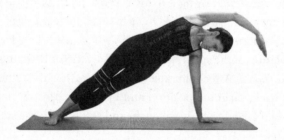

Overall goal: Strengthening the shoulders and obliques.

Postural significance: Strengthens obliques. Stretches latissimus dorsi.

Set-up: Sit facing one side with all your weight on one hip. Bend your knees slightly and place the top leg just slightly in front of the bottom leg. Place your bottom hand about six to twelve inches away from the hip, with the fingers facing away from the pelvis. Rest your top arm on your top leg.

Inhale: Lift your pelvis up off the floor and raise your top arm up towards the ceiling. Create a diagonal line with your body from the top of your head to your feet. You should have created a diagonal T shape of the body.

Exhale: Lift your pelvis up higher and bring your top arm overhead, creating a rainbow shape. Look down at your bottom hand.

Inhale: Release the rainbow shape and return to the diagonal line.

Exhale: Bend your knees and lower back down into your starting position.

Notes: Make sure the shoulders stay down and away from the ears, especially the bottom shoulder.

Repetitions: 10.

Modification: Keep your bottom leg bent with the knee on the floor beneath the hip. Keep the top leg straight out with the foot on the mat. This will reduce the pressure on the arms, shoulders and abs.

Advanced: When lowering, keep the legs straight and lower as much as possible without touching the mat, then repeat the exercise again without resting.

Basic Back Extension

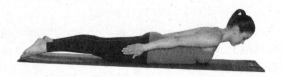

Overall goal: Strengthening the back muscles.

Postural significance: Strengthens the mid/lower trapezius. Strengthens the posterior deltoids.

Set-up: Lie face down with your forehead on the mat. Legs should be hip-width distance apart. Arms are down by the sides with the palms facing the legs.

Inhale: Visualize you are rolling a marble away with your nose. Lift the head and chest slightly off the mat keeping your eyes looking at the front edge of the mat. Squeeze the shoulder blades together at the top.

Exhale: Lower back down on the mat.

Notes: Keep the abdominals engaged and pulled into the spine. Visualize that you are lifting from the middle of the back (thoracic spine or 'lunch' portion of the back).

Repetitions: 10.

Modification: Lift the arms off the mat without lifting your head or chest. Squeeze the shoulder blades together at the top, then lower the arms back down.

Advanced: Lift your feet up off the mat at the same time as the upper body, and then lower everything back down onto the mat.

Single-Leg Kick

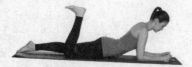

Overall goal: Strengthening all the muscles in the back, including the hamstrings.

Postural significance: Strengthens the erector spinae. Strengthens the latissimus dorsi. Stretches the abdominals.

Set-up: Lie face down and lift the upper body by placing the elbows directly beneath the shoulders, resting on your forearms. Clench the fists. Extend the legs behind you a hip-width apart. Lift the knees slightly off the mat.

Inhale: Prepare for the movement and hold.

Exhale: Bend one knee and pulse the heel towards the glute twice. Exhale twice when you pulse.

Inhale: Extend that leg back to the starting position.

Exhale: Bend the other knee and pulse the heel towards the glute twice. Exhale twice when you pulse.

Inhale: Extend the leg back to the starting position.

Notes: Keep the abdominals engaged and shoulders down and away from the ears. Use the hamstrings to lift the legs slightly off the mat. Squeeze the glutes throughout the movement.

Repetitions: 10 on each leg, alternating.

Modification: Interlace the fingers, place it under the forehead and keep the hands and head on the mat. Continue the lower body portion of the exercise.

Advanced: Flex and point the toe with each pulse of the leg towards the glute.

Double-Leg Kick

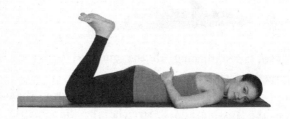

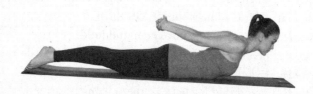

Overall goal: Strengthening all the muscles in the back of the body and stretching the chest.

Postural significance: Strengthens the erector spinae. Strengthens the latissimus dorsi. Stretches the pectorals. Stretches the abdominals.

Set-up: Lie face down and interlace the hands, bend the elbows and place the hands on the small of the back. Turn your head to one side and place that cheek on the mat. Lift the knees slightly off the mat.

Inhale: Prepare for the movement and hold.

Exhale: Bend both knees and pulse both the heels towards the glutes 3 times. Exhale 3 times when you pulse.

Inhale: Extend the legs back to the starting position, extend the arms straight behind towards the legs, keeping the hands interlaced. Lift the head, neck and shoulders off the mat and look to the front of the mat.

Exhale: Lower the upper body and turn the head to the other side. Place the hands back on the small of the back. Bend both knees and pulse both heels towards the glutes 3 times. Exhale 3 times when you pulse.

Inhale: Extend the legs back to the starting position, extend the arms straight behind towards the legs, keeping the hands interlaced. Lift the head, neck and shoulders off the mat and look to the front of the mat.

Notes: Keep the abdominals engaged, and shoulders down and away from the ears. Use the hamstrings to lift the knees slightly off the mat. Squeeze the glutes throughout the movement.

Repetitions: 5 on each side, alternating the direction the head faces (10 in total).

Modification: Interlace the fingers, place it under the forehead and keep the hands and head on the mat. Continue the lower body portion of the exercise.

Advanced: Increase to 10 repetitions on each side (20 repetitions total).

Swimming

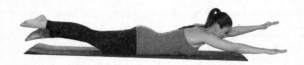

Overall goal: Strengthening all the muscles in the back of the body.

Postural significance: Strengthens the erector spinae. Strengthens the posterior deltoids.

Set-up: Lie face down and extend the arms straight up by the head. Lift the arms and knees slightly off the mat using the glutes and hamstrings to lift the legs. Keep the legs straight.

Inhale: Lift the opposite arm and opposite leg higher and alternate 5 times to a long inhale.

Exhale: Lift the opposite arm and opposite leg higher and alternate 5 times to a long exhale.

Notes: Keep the abdominals engaged and shoulders down and away from the ears. Use the hamstrings to lift the knees slightly off the mat. Squeeze the glutes throughout the movement.

Repetitions: 5 inhales and 5 exhales; 50 repetitions in total.

Modification: Keep the arms, legs and head on the mat and only lift the opposite arm and opposite leg off the mat.

Advanced: Increase to 10 inhales, 10 exhales; 100 repetitions in total.

Rocking Prep

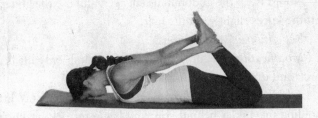

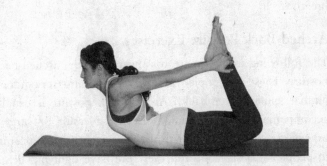

Overall goal: Strengthening all the muscles in the back of the body and stretching the chest.

Postural significance: Strengthens the erector spinae. Strengthens the posterior deltoids. Strengthens the latissimus dorsi. Stretches the pectorals.

Set-up: Lie face down, bend the knees and grab the outside of the ankles with each hand.

Inhale: Lift the head, chest and thighs off the mat. Keep your eyes looking directly forward towards the horizon.

Exhale: Lower back down to the starting position, keeping your hands on your ankles.

Notes: Keep the abdominals engaged and use the glutes to lift the knees slightly off the mat.

Repetitions: 10 repetitions.

Modification: Reduce the range of motion; only lift head, neck and upper chest off the mat.

Advanced: Perform the full rocking exercise—stay lifted holding the ankles behind you, and begin to rock backwards and forwards on the stomach by using the inhale and exhale breath.

Arched-Back Posture Exercises

The following exercises are for those with the arched-back posture. These are people with an excessive curvature in their lumbar spine (lower back). Arched-back posture is usually accompanied by weak abdominals as a result of surgery or caesarean childbirth. We also see arched-back posture in people who sit a lot and therefore have tight hip flexor muscles. (Please see Chapter 2 for a detailed description of all three postural deviations and risk factors.)

Please perform all 7 of the exercises below after you have completed your 2 warm-up exercises and 7 exercises for hunchbacks.

Rollup

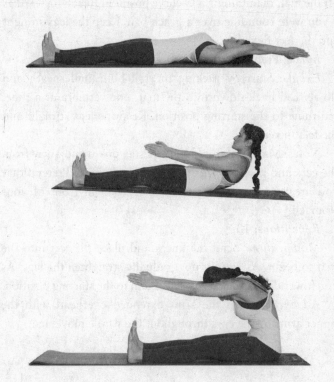

Overall goal: Stretching the spine and strengthening the abdominals.

Postural significance: Strengthens the deep intrinsic abdominals. Stretches the erector spinae.

Set-up: Lie face up with the arms extended overhead. Flex the feet by bringing the toes towards the knees.

Inhale: Lift the head, neck and shoulders off the mat and look down at the toes.

Exhale: Engage the abdominals and slowly lift the spine up off the mat, maintaining a C-curve position. Reach forward as if you were rounding over a beach ball. Keep the legs straight and the feet flexed.

Inhale: Prepare for the movement and hold.

Exhale: Start by tucking the tail bone underneath and slowly roll back down into the mat, one vertebra at a time, returning to the starting position. Keep the legs straight and the feet flexed.

Notes: Make sure the shoulders stay down and away from the ears and keep the legs planted into the mat. Pretend that you are rounding over an imaginary ball in front of your stomach.

Repetitions: 10.

Modification: Bend the knees and place the feet into the mat to begin. As you lift up, gradually straighten the legs. As you lower down, bend the knees again to the starting position.

Advanced: Keep the arms extended overhead with the upper arms by the ears throughout the whole movement.

Rolling Like a Ball

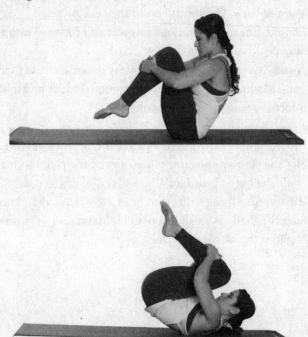

Overall goal: Stretching the spine and strengthening the abdominals.

Postural significance: Strengthens the deep intrinsic abdominals. Stretches the erector spinae.

Set-up: Sit with the knees bent and close to the chest. Wrap the arms around your legs and latch each hand onto a shin. Round the lower back, look down into the stomach and shift back slightly to balance on the glutes.

Inhale: Maintaining the position, roll backwards onto your upper back. Do not roll on to the neck or head.

Exhale: Engage the abdominals and roll forward into the starting position.

Notes: Make sure the shoulders stay down and away from the ears. Maintain the round-back position. Exhale and inhale with force to assist the movement.

Repetitions: 10.

Modification: Place the hands on the back of the thighs and let the elbows open up to the sides of the room to make the 'ball', as big as possible.

Advanced: Bring the forehead towards the knees, making the 'ball' as small as possible. Maintain this position throughout the whole exercise.

Shoulder-Bridge Prep

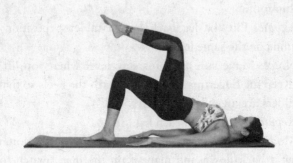

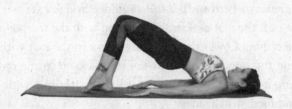

Overall goal: Strengthening the glutes and hamstrings.

Postural significance: Strengthens the glutes. Stretches the hip flexors.

Set-up: Lie face up with the knees bent and the feet placed flat on the mat. Heels should be a hip-width apart, arms by the side with the palms face down. Begin from a pelvic curl position.

Inhale: Prepare for the movement and hold.

Exhale: Lift one leg off the floor and bring it to a tabletop position with the knee over the hip and the lower leg parallel to the floor.

Inhale: Lower the leg and tap the toe on the mat. Maintain the same angle at the knee and move only from the hip joint.

Exhale: Lift the leg back into a tabletop position and continue on the same leg.

Notes: Make sure the hips stay level when you lift one leg. Keep the fingertips reaching towards the heels so that the shoulders are away from the ears.

Repetitions: 10 with each leg.

Modification: Lift one leg up to a tabletop position, then lower it back down and plant it on the mat. Switch to the other side. Alternate.

Advanced: Perform the full shoulder bridge exercise: lift one leg off the mat and straighten it up with the toe pointing to the ceiling. Lower the whole leg down to the mat without shifting the opposite hip. Lift the leg back up to the ceiling keeping it straight the whole time. Repeat 10 times with one leg and then switch sides.

Back-Support Prep

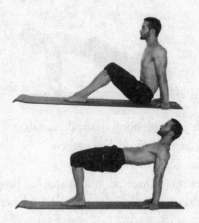

Overall goal: Strengthening the glutes and hamstrings.

Postural significance: Strengthens the glutes. Strengthens the deep intrinsic abdominals. Stretches the hip flexors.

Set-up: Sit with the legs bent and the feet flat on the mat. Place the hands behind the body with the arms straight and the fingertips facing the sides.

Inhale: Prepare for the movement and hold.

Exhale: Hinge the hips up until your torso is parallel to the ceiling. Make sure your head is aligned with your spine.

Notes: Make sure to keep the shoulders down and away from the ears.

Repetitions: Hold the position for a minimum of 20 seconds. Perform 1–3 repetitions.

Modification: Hold the position for 3 seconds each, for 8–10 repetitions.

Advanced: Sit with the legs straight and the toes pointed. Hinge the hips up until the body is in a straight line and hold.

Front Support

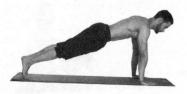

Overall goal: Strengthening the abdominals.

Postural significance: Strengthens the deep intrinsic abdominals.

Set-up: Assume a four-point kneeling-cat position with the hips directly above the knees and the shoulders directly above the wrists.

Inhale: Prepare for the movement and hold.

Exhale: Extend one leg back straight on to the ball of the foot, making sure there is no shift in the pelvis. Extend the other leg back to meet it, still keeping the pelvis stable. Create a straight line with the body from the head to the feet. Squeeze the legs and inner thighs together.

Inhale: Hold the position.

Exhale: Bend one knee back to the four-point kneeling position. Bend the other knee back into the four-point kneeling position.

Notes: Make sure the pelvis does not lift up or droop down out of alignment. Make sure the shoulders are down and away from the ears.

Repetitions: 10.

Modification: Lower the knees down to the mat and create a straight line from the head to the knees.

Advanced: Hold the extended leg position for a minimum of 30 seconds. Perform 1–3 repetitions.

Side-Lying Double-Leg Lift

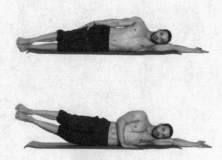

Overall goal: Strengthening the abdominals

Postural significance: Strengthens the deep intrinsic abdominals

Set-up: Lie on one side with the hips stacked directly on top of one another. Straighten the bottom arm and let the head rest on the arm. Place the top arm in front of the stomach with the palm flat on the mat. Bring the legs slightly forward from the hip joint to form a slight banana shape to the body.

Inhale: Prepare for the movement and hold.

Exhale: Lift both legs off the mat, squeezing the inner thighs and keeping the legs together.

Inhale: Back to starting position.

Exhale: Repeat the exercise.

Notes: Make sure the upper body does not lift off the mat. Use the top arm for support if needed.

Repetitions: 10.

Modification: Bring the legs further forward and let the top hip to tilt backwards, allowing the legs to lift.

Advanced: Lift the top arm up to the ceiling and do not use it for support.

Side-Kick Kneeling

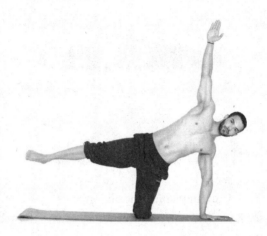

Overall goal: Strengthening the abdominals and the glutes.

Postural significance: Strengthens the deep intrinsic abdominals. Strengthens the glutes. Stretches the hip flexors.

Set-up: Kneel on both knees with the body upright and the hips directly above the shoulders. Tilt to one side and place the same arm directly under the shoulder. Extend the opposite leg out to the side, creating a diagonal line from the crown of the head to the extended toe. Lift that extended leg off the mat and hold it lifted.

Inhale: Prepare for the movement and hold.

Exhale: Bring the top leg forward for 2 pulses to 2 exhales.

Inhale: Bring the top leg backward for two pulses to two inhales.

Notes: Do not let any other part of the body move except the leg. Visualize pushing the floor away with the bottom-support hand. Make sure the shoulders (especially the bottom one) are down and away from the ears. Be sure to use the glutes when you bring your top leg to the back.

Repetitions: 10 on each side.

Modification: Perform this exercise from the side-lying leg lift position, with the whole side of the body resting on the mat and the head resting on the bottom arm. Lift the top leg and continue as described above.

Advanced: Bring the top leg forward for 2 pulses to 2 exhales and flex the foot. Bring the top leg back to 1 pulse and 1 long inhale and point the toe.

Flat-Back-Posture Exercises

The following exercises are for those with the flat-back posture. These are people who have little to no curvature in their lumbar spine, and have their tail bone tucked underneath them. This posture is also very common in those who sit all day in an incorrect position. The flat-back posture is almost always accompanied by a rounding forward of the upper body at the same time (hunchback). (Please see Chapter 2 for detailed descriptions of all three postural deviations and risk factors.)

Please perform all 7 of the exercises given below after you have completed your 2 warm-up exercises and 7 exercises for hunchback correction.

Leg Lifts

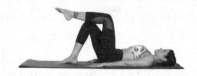

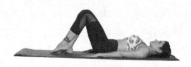

Overall goal: Strengthening the abdominals and hip flexors.

Postural significance: Strengthens the hip flexors.

Set-up: Lie face up with the knees bent and the feet flat on the mat. Heels should be hip-width distance apart. Arms by the side with the palms facing down. Pelvis should be in neutral position.

Inhale: Prepare for the movement and hold.

Exhale: Lift one leg off the mat and bring it to a tabletop position with the knee over the hip and the lower leg parallel to the mat.

Inhale: Lower the leg and touch the toe to the mat. Maintain the same angle at the knee and move only from the hip joint.

Exhale: Lift the leg back off the mat and bring it back to a tabletop position.

Notes: Engage the abdominals to keep the pelvis still throughout the movement.

Repetitions: 10 repetitions with each leg.

Advanced: Lift both legs to a tabletop position. Keep one leg in the same position while the other lowers and lifts. Complete the repetitions on one leg and switch sides.

Single-Leg Circles

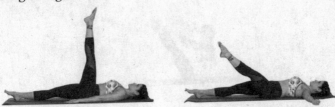

Overall goal: Strengthening the hip flexors and stretching the hamstrings.

Postural significance: Strengthens the hip flexors. Stretches the hamstrings.

Set-up: Lie face up with one leg extended straight on the mat and the other leg straight up towards the ceiling. Extend the arms out into a T position. Point both feet.

Inhale: Bring the top leg across the body, down and around to make a circle.

Exhale: Bring the top leg across the body, down and around to make a circle.

Notes: Do not let any other part of the body move except the leg, especially the opposite hip. Engage the abdominals to keep the pelvis still throughout the movement. The range of motion of the circle should be dependent on the ability to maintain a stable pelvis.

Repetitions: 10 repetitions on each leg.

Modification: Keep the top knee slightly bent and make the circle smaller.

Advanced: Perform this exercise from the shoulder-bridge position. Lift the body into a pelvic-curl position. Lift one leg straight up to the ceiling and complete a leg circle as described above.

Open-Leg Rocker

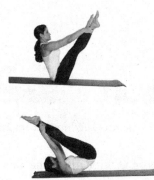

Overall goal: Stretching the back and hamstrings.

Postural significance: Strengthens the hip flexors. Stretches the hamstrings.

Set-up: Sit tall and lift one leg at a time, holding on to each ankle with each hand. Lift the chest and pull slightly on the legs to find a neutral spine. The back should be as straight as possible.

Inhale: Round the lower back and roll back to the mid-back.

Exhale: Roll forward and balance back on the glutes. Lift the chest and find neutral spine.

Notes: Make sure there is a distinct difference between the straight-back and round-back portion of the exercise. Engage the abdominals to roll back and forth.

Repetitions: 10 repetitions.

Modification: Bend the knees to a 90-degree angle and place the hands under the thighs.

Advanced: Flex the feet and hold on to the toes while performing the exercise.

Spine-Twist Sitting

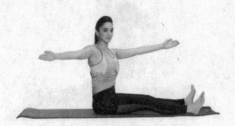

Overall goal: Strengthening the obliques and stretching hamstrings.

Postural significance: Stretches the hamstrings.

Set-up: Sit tall with the legs extended out in front, with the legs squeezed together. Arms extended out into a T position, palms face-up. Flex the feet bringing the toes towards the hips.

Inhale: Prepare for the movement and hold.

Exhale: Rotate only the upper body to one side for 2 pulses to 2 exhales.

Inhale: Return to centre.

Exhale: Rotate only the upper body to the other side for 2 pulses to 2 exhales.

Inhale: Return to centre.

Notes: Pretend that the feet are against a wall, and don't allow the feet or the pelvis to rotate. Keep the head in alignment with the spine and let it twist in the same direction as the torso. Make sure the back is as straight as possible.

Repetitions: 5 repetitions on each side (10 in total).

Modification: Bend the knees to alleviate hamstring tightness, or sit up on a yoga block to help straighten the legs.

Saw

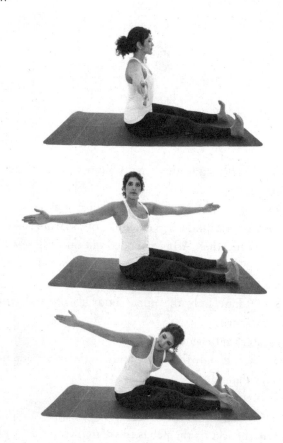

Overall goal: Strengthening the obliques and stretching the hamstrings.

   Postural significance: Stretches the hamstrings.

   Set-up: Sit tall with the legs extended out in front, wider than hip-width distance apart. Arms extended out into a T position, palms face forward. Flex the feet, bringing the toes towards the hips.

Inhale: Rotate the upper body to one side.

Exhale: Reach forward and attempt to touch the pinky finger of the front hand to the opposite toes. Allow the back arm to reach back and look backwards at the hand.

Inhale: Lift back up to the upright, rotated position.

Exhale: Return to the starting position and prepare for the other side.

Notes: When rotating to one side, attempt to keep the opposite glutes down on the mat. Visualize that the feet are against a wall and don't allow the feet or the pelvis to rotate.

Repetitions: 5 repetitions on each side (10 in total).

Modification: Bend the knees to alleviate hamstring tightness, or sit up on a yoga block to help straighten the legs.

Rollover

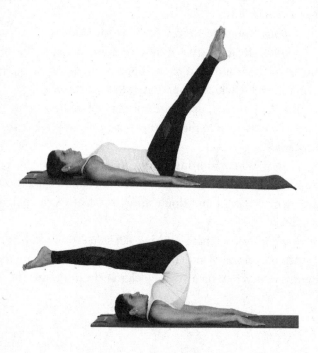

Overall goal: Strengthening the abdominals and stretching the hamstrings.

Postural significance: Stretches the hamstrings.

Set-up: Lie face-up with both legs straight up towards the ceiling. Arms should be down by the sides, palms facing down. Lower the legs down to a 45-degree angle without moving the pelvis. Point the toes.

Inhale: Lift both legs up to the ceiling.

Exhale: Lift the legs up and over the body rolling up the spine and on to the mid-back.

Inhale: Separate the legs a hip-width distance and flex the feet. Point the tail bone towards the ceiling and make sure the legs are parallel to the mat.

Exhale: Slowly lower down through the spine, one vertebra at a time. Once the legs are directly above the hips, circle them around until they meet together in the 45-degree-angle starting position.

Notes: Minimize the work of the arms and engage the abdominals when bringing the legs up and over the body. Keep the head on the mat and don't put pressure on the neck.

Repetitions: 3–5 repetitions.

Modification: Keep the knees slightly bent throughout the movement.

Advanced: When in the rollover position, attempt to touch the toes to the mat.

Corkscrew

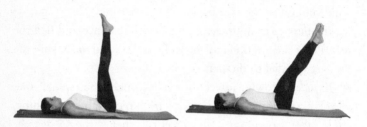

Overall goal: Strengthening the abdominals and stretching the hamstrings.

Postural significance: Strengthens the hip flexors. Stretches the hamstrings.

Set-up: Lie face up with both legs pointing straight up to the ceiling. Arms should be down by the sides, palms facing down.

Inhale: Shift both legs to one side.

Exhale: Lower the legs down and around, and complete a circle.

Inhale: Shift both legs to the other side.

Exhale: Lower the legs down and around, and complete a circle.

Notes: Do not move the upper body through the movement. The pelvis may rock to the side when the legs shift. Do not arch the lower back when the legs lower. Keep the legs together and the toes aligned.

Repetitions: 10 repetitions in total (5 in each direction).

Modification: Keep the knees slightly bent through the movement.

Advanced: Make the circle larger.

Cool-Down Exercise

The following exercise should be performed at the end of every Pilates workout.

Rolldown

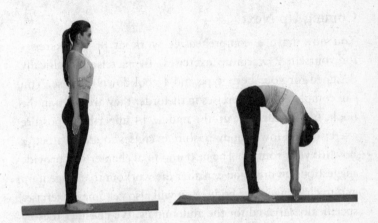

Overall goal: Stretching the back and articulating the spine.

Postural significance: Stretches the back.

Set-up: Stand with the feet a hip-width distance apart and the arms relaxed down by the sides.

Inhale: Prepare for the movement and hold.

Exhale: Lower the chin to the chest and begin to roll down the spine, bringing the arms towards the toes. Let the head and arms completely relax and be sure to keep the hips directly over the heels.

Inhale: Prepare for the movement and hold.

Exhale: Roll back up one vertebra at a time restacking the spine until upright in the starting standing position.

Notes: Keep the hips directly over the heels. Visualize rolling over a small beach ball.

Repetitions: 5 in total.

Modification: Keep the knees slightly bent through the movement.

Coming Up Next

You now have a comprehensive workout of 17 exercises for yourself: 2 warm-up exercises, 14 exercises specifically designed for your body type and 1 cool-down exercise. You can complete these exercises in the order they are given in the book, or you can mix up the middle 14 upper-body-posture exercises and lower-body-posture exercises to create a better flow for your routine. The next and final chapter will provide suggestions on how you can alter the workout to change it up and to challenge your body. You will also get 5 new exercises specifically targeted for the abdominals. We consider these 5 exercises advanced. These can be added to your routine once you have addressed any pain or postural issues you may have.

ADVANCED SHAPING TECHNIQUES

*Practice your exercises diligently with the fixed and
unalterable determination that you will permit nothing else
to sway you from keeping faith with yourself.*
Joseph Pilates, *Return to Life through Contrology*

At this point, you know your posture, you have your exercises
and you are committed to doing them daily to get in the best
shape of your life. Perhaps you have already performed some
of these exercises a few times and they are getting a bit easier.
Here are some hard-and-fast rules on how to maintain this
routine over the long haul so that your body continues to
transform into the shape of your dreams.

Change Your Body, Change Your Workout

When you perform an exercise for the first time, the muscles
are 'shocked' because they suddenly have to do things they
have never done before. They are forced to engage in a new
way for a longer period of time, or handle a heavier load
than they are used to. This means the muscle fibres actually
'break down', and when they rebuild in the subsequent days
following your workout, they rebuild stronger. This is how

Pilates and other forms of weight-bearing exercise help you to build muscles.

However, over time, your muscles become more accustomed to the same exercises and need to work less since they are now stronger and more adapted to the workout. As a result, the body no longer reflects change. The calories it takes to perform that same exercise lowers, since the muscles are stronger and the exercise is easier. For some clients who are working hard to lose weight and achieve certain goals, this can be called a 'plateau'. You can adjust your eating intake to effect a plateau like this; for instance, you can cut out more sugars, and eat more vegetables. However, it will also be essential to change up the workout and challenge your muscles in new ways. The following few paragraphs will offer a few ways to change up your routine, and to keep your body guessing and changing with your workout.

Adding Sets

Repetitions are the number of times you perform an exercise repetitively without a break. For example, you might do 10 repetitions of 'rolling like a ball' back to back without stopping. If you decide to take a break and do it again, this is considered a second 'set' of repetitions. Usually, sets are spaced with a thirty-second to one-minute break between each set. This is to give the muscles a short break to recover so that they can work hard again the second time through.

In the Pilates world, most exercises are only performed as one set. Joseph Pilates himself advised the performance of only 10 at a time.

Why Build Muscle to Lose Weight?

Have you ever met a spin or aerobics instructor who perhaps carried more weight than you imagined they would? This is quite common and is related to the 'change your workout' principle. Let's take a step aerobics instructor as an example: the first time this instructor teaches a step class, she burns 500 calories. Let's say that over time, she gets better at the workout and does it more efficiently, therefore, she now burns only 450 calories. Well, unless she adds an extra workout or cuts back on fifty calories a day of food, she will gain weight. If she isn't doing weight training or Pilates to build more muscle mass and increase her metabolism, this problem gets even worse. So alas, you will find that instructors who only teach cardio and never change their workouts will have a much harder time maintaining a slim and lean physique.

We prefer to stand by this rule, as we sincerely believe that the quality of the movement is far more important than the quantity. Therefore, if you are looking to increase the challenge of your workout, increasing the sets is an option:

- Add a second set of the exercise after a thirty-second break
- Add a challenge by repeating the whole workout from beginning to end, skipping the warm-up exercises. This would be considered the second set of the workout.

Quality versus Quantity

We say it all the time: 'The quality of the movement is far more important than the quantity of the movement.' There are many clients who brag that they can do 100 sit-ups, or 50 push-ups. However, once we get our hands on them and actually adjust their bodies to the correct position, suddenly, the exercise becomes more challenging. It's quite easy to do 100 sit-ups if you use momentum and barely lift your head. However, exercising utilizing the correct muscles and the true intrinsic core muscles makes things a whole lot more challenging. By using your core in the movement, you increase the muscle recruitment, which, in turn, burns more calories and develops more strength. So when that 'sit-up' fanatic suddenly realizes that ten very challenging sit-ups can make them sore and produce more strength than the other way, they are converts to the quality-versus-quantity mentality.

Slowing It Down

We mentioned earlier that the pace of the workout is very important, and that these exercises must not be performed with momentum. This is because slow movement, which requires the muscles to perform at their highest function, is much harder than movement that uses speed and momentum. Certain exercises like 'rolling like a ball' and 'open-leg rocker' cannot be slowed down; the momentum of rolling on the spine is necessary for proper performance of the exercise. Other exercises, such as the rollup and side bend, are made far more difficult by moving slowly. Counting to 4 in your head during each part of the exercise can assist in slowing it down and will place more load on the muscles.

Slowing it down will also increase the 'precision' of the movement. The slower you go, the more opportunity you will have to think about the muscles you are using, and ensure that your movement is coming from the correct muscles. Control is also an important principle in Pilates, and again, the movement is far more controlled the slower you go.

Pilates was adopted by many dancers in its infancy. Dancers have rhythm, therefore, the rhythm of the movements was highly influenced by the early Pilates adopters. We are not asking you to move to a beat, nor to do Pilates to fast, pounding music, but instead, to keep in mind the rhythm of the movement while performing certain exercises. If you are doing an exercise for 4 counts in one direction, do it for the same four counts back in the opposite direction. Keep the pacing the same in both directions.

Work Out with Flow

When combining the exercises described in Chapter 8, the workout can tend to be quite choppy. Some exercises are done sitting, some face down and some face up. You have a sitting exercise in the hunchback group, and a sitting exercise in the flat-back group. Why not do these back to back? Doing this can actually increase the difficulty level because it often requires you to hold yourself in the same position for a longer period of time. We have outlined two options for each possible workout combination to help increase the flow of your Pilates workout:

Hunchback/Arched-Back Workout 1

(Perform in this exact order)

Pelvic curl
Spine-stretch supine
Rollup
Rolling like a ball
Shoulder-bridge prep
Back-support prep
Spine-stretch forward
Side-lying double-leg lift
Side bend
Side-kick kneeling
Front support
Basic back extension
Single-leg kick
Double-leg kick
Swimming
Rocking prep
Rolldown

Hunchback/Arched-Back Workout 2

(Perform in this exact order)

Pelvic curl
Spine-stretch supine
Spine-stretch forward
Back-support prep
Side bend
Side-kick kneeling

Side-lying double-leg lifts
Rolling like a ball
Rollup
Shoulder-bridge prep
Basic back extension
Swimming
Rocking prep
Single-leg kick
Double-leg kick
Front support
Rolldown

Hunchback/Flat-Back Workout 1

(Perform in this exact order)

Pelvic curl
Spine-twist supine
Leg changes
Single-leg circles
Corkscrew
Rollover
Open-leg rocker
Spine-stretch forward
Spine-twist sitting
Saw
Side bend
Basic back extension
Single-leg kick
Double-leg kick
Swimming

Rocking prep
Rolldown

Hunchback/Flat-Back Workout 2

(Perform in this exact order)

Pelvic curl
Spine-twist supine
Spine-stretch forward
Spine-twist sitting
Saw
Open-leg rocker
Leg changes
Single-leg circles
Rollover
Corkscrew
Basic back extension
Single-leg kick
Double-leg kick
Rocking prep
Swimming
Side bend
Rolldown

Add More Exercises

Another way to increase the difficulty of your workout is to combine all the exercises in this book into one longer workout. This technique will increase the time you will spend doing your workout and therefore, will increase the endurance necessary for your body to perform the exercises. However, this is a sure-fire way to get into tip-top Pilates shape! This is only advised if you have addressed your postural alignment issues in Chapter 2. If you are feeling fit and strong and ready to challenge yourself, here are two workout options combining all twenty-four exercises in Chapter 8:

Full Workout 1

(Perform in this exact order)

Pelvic curl

Spine-twist supine

Leg changes

Single-leg circles

Corkscrew

Shoulder-bridge prep

Rollup

Rolling like a ball

Spine-stretch forward

Spine-twist sitting

Saw

Open-leg rocker

Rollover

Side-lying double-leg lifts

Side-kick kneeling

Side bend

Basic back extension

Double-leg kick

Single-leg kick

Swimming

Rocking prep

Front support
Back support prep
Rolldown

Full Workout 2

(Perform in this exact order)

Pelvic curl
Spine-twist supine
Rollup
Rolling like a ball
Rollover
Leg changes
Single-leg circles
Shoulder-bridge prep
Corkscrew
Open-leg rocker
Spine-stretch forward
Saw
Spine-twist sitting
Back support prep
Side bend
Side-kick kneeling
Side-lying double-leg lifts
Swimming
Rocking prep
Single-leg kick
Double-leg kick
Basic back extension
Front support
Rolldown

Bonus Abdominal Exercises

The key to adding a greater amount of challenge and progress to your workout is to add more abdominal exercises. For the most part, these exercises come from the traditional Pilates repertoire that Joseph created. We must caution you against doing some of these if you have any neck, back or spinal issues. If you are feeling strong, have been doing our Pilates workout now for at least a month and have no current pain issues, then you are ready for the following 5 exercises.

We have offered you 2 options to perform the first 4 exercises in the series: head up and head down. The head-up position requires strong abdominals. It is essential that these exercises are performed with the entire head and chest lifted off the mat, hinging from the lower ribs and looking down at the legs. It's important to avoid craning the neck up, and only using the neck muscles. At any point in this series, if the neck muscles get sore and you feel like you are not lifting with your abdominals, then please assume the head-down position for the exercise. The abdominals will still be challenged in this position.

The first of these exercises, the hundreds, is one of the exercises that defined Joseph Pilates's repertoire. It requires coordinating the arms with the breath. The final exercise in this series is the teaser. The teaser is the most challenging of all abdominal exercises in the traditional Pilates repertoire. We love that the teaser is usually placed at the end of a Pilates workout when the abdominals and spine are warmed up. Tease yourself and give it a go! And be sure to smile while you're at it.

Want an added challenge? Do these next five exercises back to back without a break.

The Hundreds

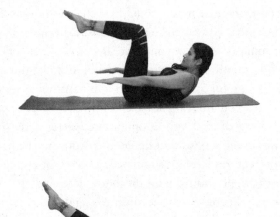

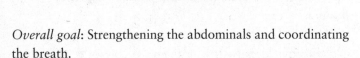

Overall goal: Strengthening the abdominals and coordinating the breath.

Set-up: Lie face up with the legs in a tabletop position, with the knees directly over the hips and the lower legs parallel to the floor. Lift the arms up and place them on the floor behind you with the upper arms parallel to the ears. Have your palms facing the ceiling.

Inhale: Prepare for the movement and hold.

Exhale: Lift the head and chest up off the floor and reach the arms down by the sides and parallel to the floor. Have your palms facing down. Look at your thighs and relax the shoulders away from the ears.

Inhale: Pump the arms up and down in small movements with 5 inhales.

Exhale: Pump the arms up and down in small movements with 5 exhales.

Notes: Keep the pelvis in a neutral position. Do not move the legs or lower body throughout the movement. Keep the breath rhythmic and controlled. Pretend that you are splashing water with your palms.

Repetitions: 100 breath repetitions in total (5 inhales, 5 exhales, 10 times).

Modification: Place the head and chest down on the mat and just pump the arms and do the breathing.

Advanced: Extend the legs straight at a 45-degree angle. Do not arch the back.

Hamstring Pull 1

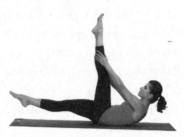

Overall goal: Strengthening the abdominals and stretching the hamstrings.

Set-up: Lie face up with the knees bent and the feet flat on the mat. Extend one leg on the mat and extend the other leg straight up towards the ceiling. Extend both hands behind the thigh (easier) or the calf (harder). Look at the thigh in front and relax the shoulders away from the ears. Keep the bottom leg firmly planted on the mat.

Exhale: Pull the top leg towards the chest gently 2 times to 2 exhales.

Inhale: Switch legs, keeping the head and chest lifted.

Exhale: Pull the top leg towards the chest gently 2 times to 2 exhales.

Notes: Keep the pelvis in a neutral position and as still as possible while switching the legs.

Repetitions: 10 repetitions total (5 with each leg).

Modification: Place the head and chest down on the mat and just lift the leg and reach behind the thigh. Continue as described above.

Advanced: Lift the bottom leg off the mat by 2 inches and never let any leg touch the mat throughout the whole exercise.

Single-Leg Stretch

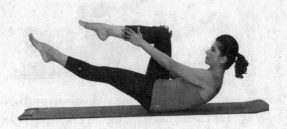

Overall goal: Strengthening the abdominals.

Set-up: Lie face up with the legs in a tabletop position, with the knees directly over the hips and the lower legs parallel to the floor. Lift the head and chest up off the floor and place both hands on one of the legs on top of the knee. Extend the opposite leg out at a 45-degree angle.

Exhale: Switch the legs, placing both hands on the opposite leg on top of the knee and extend the other leg into a 45-degree angle. Perform 2 leg switches to 2 exhales.

Inhale: Perform 2 leg switches to 2 inhales.

Notes: Keep the pelvis as still as possible while switching the legs. Don't let the pelvis rock from side to side. Don't arch the lower back.

Repetitions: 10 repetitions in total (5 with each leg).

Modification: Place the head and chest down on the mat and just perform the leg and hand movements as described above.

Advanced: Reach the arms down by the sides and keep them hovering, parallel to the floor.

Criss-Cross

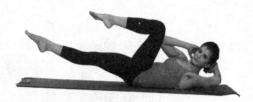

Overall goal: Strengthening the abdominals and obliques.

Set-up: Lie face up with the legs in a tabletop position, with the knees directly over the hips and the lower legs parallel to the mat. Lift the head and chest up off the floor and interlace the hands behind the head. Keep the elbows wide and the head relaxed into the hands.

Exhale: Extend one leg straight at a 45-degree angle as you rotate the upper body towards the bent knee. Pull that knee into the chest. Keep the elbows wide and rotate from the upper torso.

Inhale: Return to starting position.

Exhale: Extend the opposite leg straight at a 45-degree angle as you rotate the other side of the body towards the opposite knee. Pull that knee towards the chest. Keep the elbows wide and rotate from the upper torso.

Notes: Keep the pelvis as still as possible while switching the legs and rotating the body. Don't let the pelvis rock from side to side. Don't arch the lower back.

Repetitions: 10 repetitions in total (5 with each leg).

Modification: Keep the legs stationary in a tabletop position and rotate the upper torso side to side as described above.

Advanced: Lower the extended leg as low as it can go without arching the lower back.

Teaser

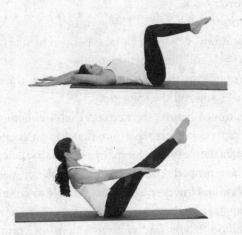

Overall goal: Strengthening the abdominals.

Set-up: Lie face up with the knees in a tabletop position, with the knees directly over the hips and the lower legs parallel to the mat. Lift the arms up behind the head with the upper arms parallel to the mat. Palms should be facing up.

Exhale: Lift your head and chest up off the mat and reach your arms towards the toes. Continue to roll the upper body up until you are balanced on the sitz bones with the back straight. Simultaneously extend both legs at a 45-degree angle in front of you.

Inhale: Prepare for the movement and hold.

Exhale: Round the lower back and begin to roll back down to the starting position keeping the legs extended at the 45-degree angle. Articulate the spine one vertebra at a time as you roll down.

Notes: Keep the shoulders away from the ears. Do not arch the lower back.

Repetitions: 5.

Modification: Bend the knees back into the tabletop position as you roll the upper torso down.

Advanced: Bring the arms up with the upper arms parallel to the ears as you roll the spine up.

As mentioned before, the above 5 exercises come directly from the Pilates classical repertoire that Joseph created years ago and often define Pilates for many enthusiasts. Being able to perform them properly can take time, consistency, persistence and motivation. However, once you are able to complete this series, you have mastered an important component of the Pilates method. If you find yourself able to perform the full teaser in a few months (with a smile), then our purpose in writing this book has been fulfilled.

CONCLUSION

*So in your very commendable pursuit of all that is implied
in the trinity of godlike attributes that only Contrology
can offer you, we bid you not good-bye but 'au revoir'
firmly linked with the sincere wish that your efforts
will result in well-merited success chained to everlasting
happiness for you and yours.*
Joseph Pilates, *Return to Life through Contrology*

It's all about you. What you put into this goal is what you will accomplish. We've given you the tools to succeed: assessment, exercises, nutrition tips and mental strategies.

First, we encourage you to do the self-assessments and take a long, hard look at your body and how it's shaped. If you work hard and do the exercises we've assigned in Chapter 8, you will achieve the body of your dreams. Adjusting your diet and becoming mindful of what you consume should also become a top priority to help you sculpt your ideal frame. We've provided some solid tips and a general framework to guide you through our recommendation of smart eating.

You also mustn't forget the other parts of your life: how you sit, stand, walk, sleep and breathe. All play an important role in achieving wellness. Shallow breathing, hunched computer work and tummy sleeping can all contribute to long-term pain and discomfort.

Most importantly, shape your attitude. Stay open-minded and take a solid look at your excuses. Look fear in the face and conquer it. Paying attention to how you stand can influence both your own emotions and how others perceive you.

Stay motivated. We are with you and wish you the best in your fitness goals now and forever.

Let Joseph Pilates have the last word: 'My work will be established and when it is, I will be the happiest man in God's Universe. My goal will have been reached.'

REFERENCES

A. Clark, Michael, C. Lucett, Scott, and G. Sutton, Brian. 2012. *NASM Essentials of Personal Fitness Training*. Baltimore: Lippincott Williams & Wilkins.

Exrx.net. 'Common Postural Deficiencies'. Available at www.exrx.net/ExInfo/Posture.html (accessed July 2014).

Jillianhessel.com. 'Who Was Joseph Pilates?' Available at www.jillianhessel.com/pilates_biography.html (accessed June 2014).

Joesplacetruepilates.com. Joseph H. Pilates: The History'. Available at www.joesplacetruepilates.com/files/2013/08/joseph-pilates1.pdf (accessed June 2014).

R. Carney, Darna, J.C. Cuddy, Amy, and J. Yapp, Andy. 2010. 'Power Posing: Brief Nonverbal Displays Affect Neuroendocrine Levels and Risk Tolerance'. *Psychological Science OnlineFirst*. Available at www0.gsb.columbia.edu/mygsb/faculty/research/pubfiles/4679/power.poses_.PS_.2010.pdf (accessed October 2014).

Shahul Hameed, P. July 2013. 'Prevalence of Work Related Lower Back Pain Among the Information Technology Professionals In India: A Cross Sectional Study'. *International Journal of Scientific and Technology Research* (2: 7). Available at www.ijstr.org/final-print/july2013/Prevalance-Of-Work-Related-Low-Back-Pain-

Among-The-Information-Technology-Professionals-In-India---A-Cross-Sectional-Study.pdf.

Thomson, Bruce. 'Biography of Joseph Hubertus Pilates'. Easyvigour.net. Available at www.easyvigour.net.nz/pilates/h_biography.htm (accessed June 2014).

ACKNOWLEDGEMENTS

They say it often takes a village, and in this case, it definitely took one to get this book into print.

First and foremost, we would both like to thank our parents, who gave us abundant love and helped us grow up to be independent, confident people.

Next, we thank Gurveen Chadha, Milee Ashwarya and the team at Penguin Random House for their trust, faith and endless support. What an amazing experience it has been to work with them!

A huge thank you goes to Thom Meyer for endless hours of editing, and to Kim Meyer for her love and support through those hours of editing.

To Jennifer Pearlstein, Ann Toran, Nora St John, Rael Isacowitz and Kathy Mulherin for being trusted advisors and mentors. A special thank you goes to Jennifer and Kathy for reading and evaluating this book at a critical time.

Another special thank you from Yasmin to Sensei Pervez Mistry for being her mentor, her inspiration and the essence of who she is. A special shout-out to my brother, Saif Qureishi, for being my advisor and guide, and always pushing me to do better and go further. Another special thanks to my in-laws, for moving into my house for three months to look after my sons so that I could go and learn how to teach Pilates.

Thank you, Linda Joseph-Turek from Silver Moon Photography, for Zeena's pictures. Thank you, Jean Kapcio and Falisha Kurji, for assisting in the photo shoot. To my clients and friends at Vertical Pilates: You inspire me on a daily basis.

A thank you to Munna S. for Yasmin's photography, to Ashley Rebello for styling her shoot, and to Luluaa Mathias for her make-up and for that of the models. A thank you to Nishreen Kanchwala for being the person behind the scenes at all my shoots. A special thanks to team Body Image for bearing with my absence and my mood swings, and always encouraging me. I'm most grateful to all my clients, past and present, for trusting me on their journey to getting fitter. Without them, this wouldn't have been possible. A special shout-out to my friend Resham Lalwani, who patiently allows me to experiment on her whenever I have a new workout that I want to perfect. Thank you, all my friends, for getting excited at my every accomplishment.

A thank you to our wonderful models: Waluscha De Sousa, Anita Raj, Kiara Advani, Falisha Kurji and Sahib for adding spice to the book. A thank you to Bryan Weissman for working on the graphics.

To our husbands, Azeem Dhalla and Minhaz Karachiwala: Thank you both for your patience and for tolerating our endless Skype calls at odd hours. You are our rocks of Gibraltar. Without you, we could not have pursued our dreams.

To our children, Zahaan, Amaan and Zaleeya. You are our inspiration. Dream big! To Yasmin's beloved nieces, Shaazia and Aaliyah. We love you!

A giant thank you for your gracious testimonials, Salman Khan, Deepika Padukone, Katrina Kaif, Kareena Kapoor, Alia Bhatt, Ileana D'Cruz, Imran Khan, Jennifer Pearlstein, John Gloster, Karan Johar, Kiara Advani, Kinita Kadakia Patel, Kristofer McNeeley, Kunal Kapoor, Malaika Arora Khan, Michelle Dube, Preity Zinta, Rhea Pillai, Ridham Desai, Sophie Choudry, Zaheer Khan, Zareen Khan, Evelyn Sharma and Zoya Akhtar.

A NOTE ON THE AUTHORS

Yasmin Karachiwala is amongst the most well known of Mumbai's fitness professionals. She is the founder and director of Body Image, a personal training fitness studio located in Bandra. Her journey into the world of health and fitness began with her own discovery of her level of fitness over twenty-two years ago, and since then, she has committed her professional life to promoting health, fitness and overall quality of life. A mother of two, she is a role model for youngsters and adults alike. She practises what she preaches, and is extremely fit herself. Her credo has always been about not just looking good, but also feeling good, and being healthy and energetic.

Yasmin's skill set is broad and deep. She is the only Balanced Body® Master Trainer in India, certified faculty for Mat, Reformer, CoreAlign and Motr. She is also the only BASI (Body Arts and Science International)-certified Pilates instructor in India, and specializes in mat work as well as the utilization of different machines (Reformer, Cadallac, CoreAlign, Wunda Chair, etc.). She has trained in many institutions globally, and on an ongoing basis, stays abreast of emerging principles in the world of fitness. Her approach towards promoting fitness and health includes not just weight loss, but also improvement of posture, coordination, strength, flexibility and endurance. She believes that a body that performs well bio-mechanically, automatically functions more efficiently, burns more fat and performs better overall.

At Body Image, Yasmin uses a variety of modalities and equipment for fitness training. Her focus is on individual assessments and designing highly-customized fitness programmes for each member based on their requirements, goals, likes, dislikes, and body type.

She is highly respected in fitness circles, and her advice is frequently solicited. She was the official fitness expert for the Pantaloons Femina Miss India 2011 contest, and trained all of the contestants. She has made a multitude of appearances on television, including being a jury member on *Get Gorgeous* and featuring in an NDTV fitness show with Kim Sharma. She has also appeared regularly in the print media *(Mother and Baby, TIMES OF INDIA – ROUGE, Hi! Blitz)*, and as a talk show guest on Fitness Radio FM 93.7. She has written multiple articles for newspapers and magazines like *Bombay Times*, *Mumbai Mirror* and *Vogue*.

She is a well-known name and an extremely sought-after fitness expert in Bollywood circles. Her personal training clientele include high-profile individuals such as Katrina Kaif, Kareena Kapoor, Karishma Kapoor, Deepika Padukone, Alia Bhatt, Sohail Khan, Malaika Arora Khan, Bipasha Basu, Sonakshi Sinha, Sonam Kappor, Ileana D'cruz, Preity Zinta, Imran Khan, Kunal Kapoor, Zoya Akhtar, Anita Raaj, Neha Dhupia, Arjun Rampal, Mehr Jesia, Zareen Khan, Yuvraj Singh, Ajit Agarkar and Zaheer Khan.

* * *

Zeena Dhalla is a premier personal trainer and Pilates instructor in Orange County. She is the founder of Vertical Pilates, the first vertical-only Pilates studio in the US. Zeena graduated with a degree in communications from Northwestern University, one of the top-ranked universities in the US. Her fitness education includes her Pilates course from BASI (Body Arts and Sciences International) where she received certifications in mat, Reformer, Trapeze Table, Wunda Chair and Ladder Barrel. She has her personal training certification from NASM (National Academy of Sports Medicine), and her CoreAlign certification from Balanced Body University. She has also completed coursework in integrative flexibility from NASM, and is a trained wellness coach. She has recently been certified as a postural specialist from the National Posture Institute.

Zeena has worked for years as a mentor and instructor for many fitness professionals, having served as a manager in the fitness industry for many years. She was the owner and operator of the Athletic Club for Women, in Newport Beach, California, where she grew the Pilates programme there by over 200 per cent during her ownership period. She then went on to serve as Pilates director for the Orange County division of YogaWorks, the premier Pilates and yoga studio in Orange County. She has taught courses in sales and business development for fledgling fitness professionals.

Zeena has been featured as a writer and fitness model by *OC Squeeze, OC Metro, OC Register,* and on the television show *Daybreak OC*. She was recently featured in *Pilates Style* magazine as the author and model for *Pilates for Baby Boomers*. Zeena has served on the board of directors for the National Association for Women Business Owners. Her philanthropic responsibilities include fundraising for organizations such as HelpUsAdopt.org, Relay for Life Cancer, and A Little Bit of Sunshine (that funds orphanages in India and Nepal).

Since becoming a mom to her daughter (she and her husband adopted from Kolkata in 2008), Zeena has focused on maintaining the balance between work and motherhood. Her clients love her for being tough and demanding on their form, but gentle and encouraging in her coaching. She believes that fitness is far more than fitting into a tight pair of pants, and that achieving wellness starts from within. 'No self-deprecating talk' is the motto in her studio, and she wants everyone to walk out feeling stronger, leaner and, most importantly, more confident in themselves.